Food Chaining

Food Chaining

The Proven 6-Step Plan to Stop Picky Eating, Solve Feeding Problems, and Expand Your Child's Diet

Cheri Fraker, CCC/SLP,
Laura Walbert, CCC/SLP, Sibyl Cox, LD, RD
and Mark Fishbein, MD
with Shannon Cole Barker, OTR/L

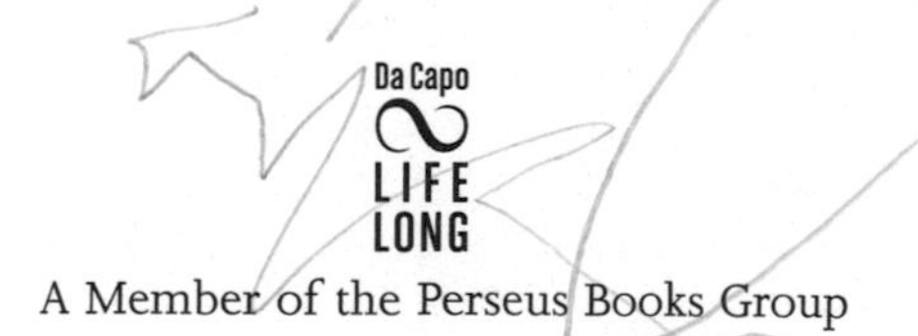

A Member of the Perseus Books Group

Many of the designations used by manufacturers and sellers to distinguish their products are claimed as trademarks. Where those designations appear in this book and Da Capo Press was aware of a trademark claim, the designations have been printed in initial capital letters.

 Printed in the United States of America. For information, address Da Capo Press, 11 Cambridge Center, Cambridge, MA 02142.

Designed by Maria E. Torres
Set in 12 point AGaramond by the Perseus Books Group

Cataloging-in-Publication data for this book is available from the Library of Congress.

ISBN: 978-1-60094-016-3

Published by Da Capo Press
A Member of the Perseus Books Group
www.dacapopress.com

Note: The information in this book is true and complete to the best of our knowledge. This book is intended only as an informative guide for those wishing to know more about health issues. In no way is this book intended to replace, countermand, or conflict with the advice given to you by your own physician. The ultimate decision concerning care should be made between you and your doctor. We strongly recommend you follow his or her advice. Information in this book is general and is offered with no guarantees on the part of the authors or Da Capo Press. The authors and publisher disclaim all liability in connection with the use of this book. The names and identifying details of people associated with events described in this book have been changed. Any similarity to actual persons is coincidental.

Da Capo Press books are available at special discounts for bulk purchases in the U.S. by corporations, institutions, and other organizations. For more information, please contact the Special Markets Department at the Perseus Books Group, 2300 Chestnut Street, Suite 200, Philadelphia, PA, 19103, or call (800) 810-4145, extension 5000, or e-mail special.markets@perseusbooks.com.

10 9 8 7 6 5

This book is dedicated to Maria Batten, and to Eliot Batten,
"The Father of Food Chaining,"
and to all our patients and their wonderful families.

Contents

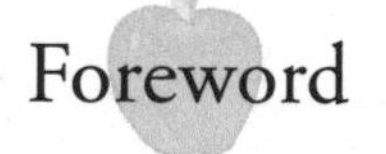

Foreword

AS AN OCCUPATIONAL therapist who works with children with feeding issues, I've had many parents share with me how lost, defeated, and disappointed they feel as a result of caring for a child with feeding difficulties. These parents feel they are to blame for their children's feeding problems and that they have failed them. By the time their children have enrolled in therapy, the parents are usually filled with guilt and emotionally exhausted. The truth is that your child's picky or problem eating is not your fault, and you have done the best you can for your child given the resources available to you. Now there is a new resource available: it's called *food chaining*.

The vast majority of children with a feeding disorder have a medical condition, an oral motor skills problem, a sensory processing disorder, a behavioral issue, or some combination thereof that is affecting their ability to eat. As an occupational therapist, I specialize in the sensory aspects of a feeding problem. My role is to establish what I call a child's "sensory framework" by evaluating her five senses as they relate to feeding. During the evaluation process, I identify how a child orients, processes, and registers sensory information (i.e., the appearance, smell, taste, and texture of the food) when she is eating. This is crucial information, because it gives me a clear and concise picture of a child's sensory tolerance to particular foods. More important, it helps me uncover a pattern that explains why the child accepts certain foods and rejects others (her sensory framework).

Food chaining is so effective because, unlike other feeding therapies, it takes all the child's sensory framework senses into account and it deals with the sensory challenges many children with feeding problems face. This specialized feeding therapy uses a team of medical experts (also known as a feeding team) to evaluate your child and determine exactly where the feeding process is breaking down for her. You will learn to understand how your child perceives the appearance, texture, smell, and taste of food, and why she reacts the way she does. With this knowledge, you and your child's feeding team will create a step-by-step treatment program to help her overcome her feeding problems. You will first establish a list of her preferred, tolerated, and rejected foods and gradually expand her diet safely and naturally based on her personal sensory tolerance and her emotional comfort.

One of the greatest strengths of food chaining is that the program is driven not just by the child, but by the parents and the needs of the entire family. The program is built around your goals for your child, whether they are to introduce your child to fruits and vegetables or to eat a meal as a family without confrontation or meltdowns. It is implemented by you at home with the support of the feeding team.

Whatever your goal may be, it can be achieved if you recognize and appreciate that there are numerous sensory influences on your child along the way. Food chaining is a wonderful program that can either complement your child's current treatment plan or offer crucial guidance if you are seeking help in overcoming your child's picky or problem eating. I commend Cheri Fraker, Laura Walbert, Sibyl Cox, and Dr. Mark Fishbein for their dedication to feeding therapy. I thank them for inviting both parents and professionals working in the "world of feeding" to apply food chaining to our current regimen of treatment.

Shannon Cole Barker, OTR/L
Pediatric Occupational Therapist

Introduction

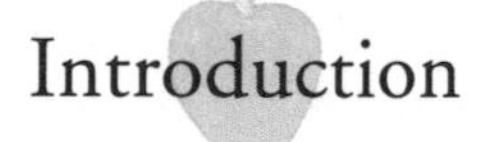

Sam was a beautiful baby, the kind of child that every mother pictures in her head when she discovers she is expecting. He was born in perfect health, always seemed to be in a good mood, slept well, and sailed through all the stages of development until he turned one year old, when his parents decided to make the jump to table foods. It seemed as if Sam woke up one day and forgot how to eat. When his mother, Christi, gave him a Cheerio, Sam just held the cereal in his mouth, not chewing it. Christi could see it sitting on the back of his tongue. Then he started gagging and crying. It scared Sam and it scared Christi.

Whenever Christi offered Sam any table food, he turned his face away from the spoon or batted it away with his hands. Christi knew that it often takes kids several tries before they'll accept a new food, but no matter how many times she offered a food, Sam would never eat it. In desperation, Christi went back to baby food, but Sam didn't really seem to want that, either. He pushed the spoon away from his mouth. All he wanted was to drink his milk. At every meal he sat in his high chair and cried until Christi got him out and gave him his bottle. Christi had heard that most kids go through a picky eating stage, but Sam's food refusals didn't seem normal to her. She worried that his limited diet was harming him, but she didn't know how to get him to try new foods. Christi realized that the time had come for her to get some help for Sam.

AS PARENTS, WE face many difficult challenges as we try to raise happy, healthy children. One of the biggest challenges is helping our kids learn to be good eaters. We all want our kids to eat nutritious foods from a wide variety of sources in the proper portion sizes. We do our best to prepare appealing and well-balanced meals for our kids and show them how to make smart food choices. But eating the right foods, or even eating at all, is not so easy for some children. Between 25 and 35 percent of children in the United States are considered picky or problem eaters. This statistic becomes even higher—between 40 and 70 percent—for children with chronic medical problems. Parents are often told, "It's just a stage, he'll grow out of it," or, "He'll eat if he gets hungry enough," but picky eating and problem eating, also known as feeding disorders, are serious concerns. They can cause medical problems such as malnutrition, frequent illness, and congestion. They can affect your child's development in areas such as growth and weight gain. They can negatively impact your child's behavior. Feeding disorders can also interfere with his social skills and his ability to concentrate and learn at school.

Your child isn't the only one affected. Living with a picky or problem eater is stressful for the entire family. "Every meal is like a battle. I constantly try, but my son won't try anything new or eat any food that isn't on his list of favorites. It drives me and my husband crazy, and we often wind up taking out our frustrations on the kids. The whole family is usually miserable by the end of each meal," says Jill. Many parents report extreme stress at mealtimes. Problems with eating often start in infancy, and these problems must be faced multiple times every day, with every meal. So it's no surprise that mealtimes can become anxiety-driven experiences or constant battles that involve everyone at the table. You may be feeling anxious about your child's nutrition and growth. You may feel angry and frustrated by the way he's behaving. You may be having doubts about yourself or your parenting abilities. You may even be feeling depressed about your child's situation and your apparent inability to fix it. These negative feelings can easily spill over into other areas of your life, such as the workplace or your relationships with others. Your relationship with your child may also be suffering. Feeding problems can cause children to withdraw or act out. You may find that you're constantly arguing with your child over eating and the way he's behaving. One mother told us that her child's feeding problems made her life feel like "a train that has derailed."

Siblings are also affected by the stress of living with a picky or problem eater. Some parents (understandably so) spend so much of their time and energy focusing on getting their child to eat or managing his behavior that the needs of their other children get overlooked. It's so easy to become angry and frustrated by their picky or problem eater and unconsciously take that stress out on the rest of the family. Meals and family time in general become unhappy and toxic for everyone.

You may find that your relationship with your partner is suffering, as well. The constant stress caused by your child's feeding problems can create tension between you. You may not agree on the right way to handle mealtimes with your child or the best way to manage his behavior, which can lead to arguments and bad feelings.

Clearly, picky and problem eating are major issues that affect a huge number of children, yet they are still widely overlooked problems in the medical field. A child can be at an appropriate weight, but poorly nourished. Many picky and problem eaters appear well nourished and thrive despite their feeding problems (some are even overweight), which can make health-care practitioners reluctant to address the issue. It's not unusual for health-care practitioners to tell concerned parents that their children will "grow out" of their feeding difficulties. Many times this is simply not the case. Based on our experience as a feeding team and as medical professionals who work with children, we can tell you that your child's eating issues will probably not resolve themselves on their own, and it's unlikely that can you solve this problem without help. Feeding issues are very complex—they can have health-related, physical, sensory, or psychological causes, or a combination thereof—and it takes the expertise of several different types of medical professionals to determine the nature of your child's problem and design a treatment program for him. *Food Chaining* will help you navigate this process so your entire family can live happier, healthier lives.

IS YOUR CHILD A PICKY EATER OR A PROBLEM EATER?

Sometimes it can be difficult to tell if a child is a picky eater, has a more serious feeding problem, or is just behaving as normal children do when it comes to food. Most parents expect a certain amount of resistance and fussiness from their kids over food and mealtimes. For your convenience, we've listed below the criteria for normal, picky, and problem eaters. This will help you differentiate among the terms and determine into which category your child falls.

NORMAL EATERS

Following is an at-a-glance guide to normal eating behaviors and skills for newborns through age two.

Newborn Baby to Three Months A typical newborn baby consumes 2 ounces (or 60 milliliters) of formula in as little as about 5 minutes up to 20 minutes. At this age, your baby may not completely coordinate sucking and breathing at first.

Three Months At this age, your baby should sequence 20 or more sucks from the breast or bottle, and breathing should follow sucking with no pauses when he is hungry. Your baby should be able to coordinate pauses for breathing. You may observe an occasional cough if his coordination of the suck/swallow/breathe sequence becomes irregular. He still does not have the skills to start baby food.

Four to Six Months Now your baby should use long sequences of sucking, swallowing, and breathing when breast- or bottle-feeding. His tongue should show an extension-retraction pattern of tongue movement, or a forward and then backward movement. If you start your baby on a spoon now, he is likely to push it out due to the continued presence of the **tongue protrusion reflex.** It is best to wait until closer to six months to introduce a spoon.

Cup Skills Many parents are instructed to introduce a sippy cup to their child at age six months. However, this does not mean that your child should be expected to take all liquids by cup. Some children do not demonstrate good cup skills until 9 or 10 months of age, and still others don't become adept at cup drinking until 12 to 15 months. Your baby may continuously suck liquid from the cup and then have periods of uncoordinated swallowing. He may lose much of the liquid while drinking. Larger mouthfuls may result in choking or coughing.

Six Months At six months your baby should develop a more mature sucking pattern. His jaw movement should decrease and his lips should more firmly surround the nipple or spoon.

Your baby is now ready to accept thicker consistencies of food. His tongue protrusion reflex should be integrated, and he should no longer push food out of his mouth with his tongue. When eating meals, your baby may need more support for his body, such as rolled towels wedged on either side of him when he's seated in his high chair.

Nine Months At this age, your baby should exhibit long sequences of continuous sucks when cup drinking, though he may still have coordination issues with the cup. Usually at this age babies can take three sucks or so before pulling away to breathe. When spoon-feeding, you may see a munching style (up-and-down sucking pattern) on the spoon, but a more mature pattern of chewing should be emerging. You may also see his tongue protrude between his teeth or gums. He should be stable while sitting by this point and no longer need additional support for his body.

Nine to Twelve Months You may still see occasional mild coughing when your baby drinks from his cup. He should be able to lateralize his tongue more efficiently now (move it to the side of the mouth). He should be able to take a controlled bite of a soft cookie. He may suckle on a harder cookie or food to soften it prior to taking a bite.

Twelve to Fifteen Months At this age, your baby should have a well-coordinated suck/swallow/ breathe sequence, and only rare coughing or choking spells should occur. Your baby should be able to suck food off a spoon. Your baby should be developing a pincer grasp and beginning to master self-feeding. He should be able to hold his own cup. Your baby should be able to handle a variety of textures of food by age 15 months.

Eighteen Months You should no longer see an extension-retraction pattern (a forward and then backward movement) of your child's tongue with a spoon. He should have a more mature pattern of chewing where food is pushed from the tongue to the biting surfaces and moved back to the tongue to prepare for swallowing. Your child should have good lip closure while chewing and not lose food when eating. He should be able to take a controlled bite of a hard cookie. You may notice that your child moves his arms or legs while biting or tips his head back slightly to assist with the bite. At this point your child should have excellent hand-to-mouth skills and may be able to drink from a straw.

Twenty-Four Months Your child should be able to drink well from a cup or straw. He should be able to skillfully swallow a combination of food textures. He should exhibit controlled biting patterns and be able to keep his head in a midline position while biting into food.

Children Over Age Two Your child should continue to improve and refine his eating skills during the years of early childhood. He should master the ability to manipulate all types of food easily in his mouth and develop very sophisticated chewing skills by age six. By this point, your child should be able to eat even the hardest-to-eat foods, such as taffy and all types of meat.

Picky Eaters

- A picky eater is very selective about what foods he will eat.
- A picky eater accepts 30 or more foods.
- A picky eater will want to eat certain foods for many days at a time.
- If a picky eater tires of a food and stops eating it, he will usually accept the food again after a break from eating it.

Picky eaters generally don't have a medical condition but they may have had reflux as an infant or a milder underlying sensory issue that prevents them from eating certain foods. They often become picky because they've been exposed to only a few foods and have developed food preferences based on a cycle of limited exposure. However, picky eaters can experience true distress at meals as well.

Three-year-old Emma is a good example of a picky eater. Her mother, Cara, says that Emma ate very well during her first year of life. She ate all her fruits, vegetables, and meat baby foods until she was well past her first birthday. When she was 15 months old, her mother tried to transition her from stage III baby foods to table foods. (Babies foods come in stages based on a baby's age and eating abilities. All babies begin at age four to six months with stage 1 foods, which are single ingredient foods like rice cereal and pureed fruits and vegetables. At seven to eight months of age, babies begin eating stage 11 foods, which consist of single ingredient and combination foods that are strained instead of pureed. At nine to twelve month of age, babies are ready for stage 111 foods, which have more texture and contain chunks to help encourage chewing.) Emma slowly made the transition, but she was very selective with table foods and would only eat particular brands or food from particular restaurants. One day Cara offered Emma macaroni and cheese, which she ate very well, and Cara was thrilled. For a long time after that it seemed that macaroni and cheese was the only food Emma ever wanted. Then one day she stopped accepting it and refused it each time it was offered. Cara says that this became a pattern with Emma. She would eat one "favorite" food for a long time and then reject it. Emma eventually tried the food again, but it never again became the favorite food it was when she first accepted it.

Problem Eaters

- A problem eater accepts only a few foods, usually fewer than 20.
- A problem eater may have a strong phobic reaction to new foods. He may cry, throw a tantrum, gag, or vomit when a new food is offered.
- A problem eater may not even be able to touch new foods.

- If a food is rejected after eating it for an extended time, a problem eater has a hard time accepting the food again.
- A problem eater may reject entire groups of food (i.e., he won't eat any vegetables or any fruits at all).

Problem eaters usually have some type of medical condition, such as **GERD** (a condition where a child experiences recurrent vomiting or spitting up as well as other possible symptoms, which are discussed in chapter 1) or oral motor skill problems, that prevents them from eating certain foods. A problem eater may also have a sensory processing disorder or food aversion, meaning they may gag or vomit at the sight or touch of food.

Two-year-old Jack is a good example of a problem eater. His mother, Amy, says eating has always been difficult for Jack. As a baby, he had to work hard to finish his bottles. He struggled with the transitions to spoon and cup. He never seems hungry. He doesn't appear to have a choking problem, but he never seems to enjoy eating. Meals are always a struggle. Every new food Amy offers seems to cause Jack distress. He appears to be almost afraid of food. After Jack moved to table foods, he became more and more selective, and now his diet consists of only five "junk" foods. Amy is very worried about nutrition because Jack will not eat fruits, vegetables, or meats. Each time she offers these foods, Jack gags, cries, and refuses to eat.

Regardless of where your child falls in the categories listed above, if you find yourself short-order cooking for your child, if food items are dropping out of his diet, or if mealtime battles are a regular occurrence, it's time to discuss these concerns with his pediatrician and have him evaluated.

HOW TO USE THIS BOOK

We wrote *Food Chaining* as a tool to help as many children with eating problems as possible. In order to do this most effectively, we have detailed how the food-chaining program works in its entirety. Not every child will need to see every health professional or go through every step that we describe in this book, but some will. For instance, kids who have a milder picky-eating issue may not need to see a nutritionist. Kids who suffer from a feeding disorder caused by a medical condition may not need to see a behavioral psychologist. On the other hand, a child with a serious feeding disorder will almost certainly need to follow every step in the food-chaining program. It will be up to you and your child's pediatrician to determine the extent of your child's program based on his needs. Regardless of where your child falls on the spectrum of eating problems, there is valuable information in each of these chapters that will help you understand how your child interacts with food, as well as strategies to help him become more comfortable with food and improve his diet.

As eating problems can begin at any age and last indefinitely if left untreated, *Food Chaining* is designed to help children from birth through early adulthood. If you have an infant less than one year of age, he may qualify for the pre-chaining program we describe in chapter 7.

Food Chaining was written specifically for the parents and caregivers of picky and problem eaters. However, the information and strategies offered in these pages will also be helpful for parents who wish to help their kids avoid potential feeding problems and medical professionals who work with children with feeding problems. Though we've kept our use of medical terms to the absolute minimum, you may come across some that are unfamiliar to you. For easy reference, we've provided a glossary of these terms and they are printed in **boldface** the first time they appear in the book.

WHAT IS FOOD CHAINING?

Food chaining was created by Cheri Fraker in the course of treating an 11-year-old boy named Eliot. Eliot's problems with food started at age 18 months, when he began demonstrating a pattern of picky eating, and more and more foods dropped out of his diet. By the time he reached childhood, his diet consisted only of peanut butter, white bread, and large quantities of milk. He refused to try any new foods, and was very sensitive to the smell of meat.

Eliot did not "grow out" of his picky eating, as his mother was told he would. In fact, a very complex feeding disorder had developed out of what began as picky eating. When Eliot was evaluated by Cheri and the rest of the feeding team, they determined that he was taking in such a large quantity of milk that he was anemic. Although his weight was appropriate, he was poorly nourished. Eliot's feeding problem had also begun to affect his social life. His mother reported that when Eliot was invited to a sleepover or a birthday party, food was always an issue. Eliot wanted to go to a two-week summer camp but couldn't, because he would be facing 18 meals that did not consist of peanut butter, white bread, and milk. Cheri and the team discussed the future impact of Eliot's selective eating and the limits it would place on his social life, including dating, and came up with a program they thought would help.

Eliot started weekly therapy sessions with Cheri. One day during a session Eliot said to Cheri, "Do you know that pizza and spaghetti taste kind of the same?" Cheri said that she did know that, but it struck her that Eliot *didn't* know that. She wondered what would happen if she started grouping foods that appealed to him by taste and teaching him about food. Eliot was so far behind in his exposure to foods, Cheri decided to try it.

She asked him to rate pizza sauce and spaghetti sauce on a scale from 1 to 10, and thereafter they kept on rating different foods. Cheri kept track of all of Eliot's ratings and noticed, a few weeks later, how much higher the ratings were for foods after he had tried them several times. Pizza went from a 4 to a 10 in about five weeks.

Cheri continued selecting specific foods for Eliot based on what he enjoyed eating. He made rapid improvement in treatment and went from 5 foods to 150 in three months. Pizza became his favorite food. There were still foods he didn't like, and he was encouraged to express himself if he did not want to try certain foods. The goal was never to get Eliot to eat every food. The goal was to help him find foods he liked in each food group. At the end of treatment, Eliot had a balanced diet and was able to find something to eat in any restaurant or social situation. Over the course of his one year of treatment, his nutritional status improved greatly, and he met all his treatment goals, including a successful two weeks at camp. Eliot would always have favorite foods, and that was just fine. His family was cautioned that there would likely be some regression when the therapy came to an end. It was not an easy or a quick fix, but Eliot and his family were committed to the program, and Eliot was motivated to change his eating patterns. He has maintained his healthy eating habits and today he is a thriving 15-year-old.

Feeding problems can be very complex and are usually caused by a combination of factors. Some children have problems that begin at birth with breast- or bottle-feeding. These infants may have difficulty controlling liquid in the mouth or may have a swallowing problem that allows them to take in only small amounts of liquid at a time. Some children have medical problems such as gastroesophageal reflux or food allergies that contribute to their food refusal. Still other kids have sensory issues that cause them to find entire food groups impossible to tolerate. It's not uncommon for these children to gag when looking at or touching food. Regardless of the source of the problem, what's clear is that once a child learns that eating is uncomfortable in some way, he will start to avoid it.

This is where the food-chaining program comes in. *Food Chaining* presents a six-step treatment plan developed specifically to help kids overcome feeding problems and expand their diet safely and naturally.

The first five steps of the program are designed to determine the reasons your child is refusing to eat. We'll help you to examine every aspect of your child's eating habits and skills, and to evaluate him to see if his eating issues are medical or sensory-based problems. The first step is always to take your child to his pediatrician for a medical exam. We then recommend that your child see other members of a "feeding team," typically a **pediatric dietitian,** a pediatric speech therapist, an occupational therapist, and a behavioral psychologist. Each of these professionals can assess your child and pool their findings in order to get a complete picture of your child's picky or problem eating. Your pediatrician may work with or be able to refer you to a feeding team in your area. The following is a rundown of the steps.

- Step 1 will help you determine if your child has an underlying medical condition, such as a digestive disorder, that's contributing to his feeding problem.
- Step 2 will help your child get the nutrition he needs and help you figure out if food allergies are playing a role. Good nutrition is critical for all children—it plays a key role in brain and bone growth and supports their ability to fight infection and viruses. But it's particularly important for picky eaters, as they are at greater risk for nutritional problems.
- Step 3 will guide you through oral motor skill problems that may affect your child's ability to eat, such as chewing or swallowing difficulties.

- Step 4 will help you understand how your child handles sensory input and why he may react to food the way he does. Our senses play a very important role in our ability and willingness to eat. Kids with a **sensory processing disorder** or **feeding aversion** have a negative response to the taste and texture of some or all foods.
- Step 5 offers strategies for handling your child's negative mealtime behaviors. Your child's behavior offers many clues to the nature of his eating problems. You'll also learn strategies for teaching your child about food, which is a key part of this program.

Once the experts have weighed in and a feeding program has been created based on your child's individual needs, it's time to start food chaining.

The concept behind step 6, the food-chaining solution, is simple. There are very specific reasons why your child will only eat certain foods. There is something about these foods (it could be the texture, the flavor, the temperature, or even just the look of them) that your child finds acceptable. Food chaining determines why your child accepts these certain foods. Then, you can begin to expand his food repertoire by introducing to him new foods that have the same features as the foods he currently eats. Once your child has expanded the foods he will eat in this way, you can introduce new foods with slightly different tastes or textures.

For example, Lisa was concerned that her five-year-old

daughter, Emily, wasn't getting enough nutrition, since she'd eat only oatmeal, pudding, or yogurt for dinner. It turned out that Emily was highly sensitive to foods that changed during the process of chewing from one texture to another. She preferred to eat very simple foods with strong flavors. To help her move beyond her texture sensitivities, we developed a program introducing new foods that had a smooth, creamy texture Emily could tolerate. The next step will be adding some slight texture to her accepted foods to help her expand her diet.

Slowly but surely, you'll continue to expand your child's food repertoire until he is consistently eating a healthy, balanced diet with a wider taste or texture preference. While food-chaining programs are generally designed by a speech therapist with the assistance of a pediatric dietitian, occupational therapist, and behavioral psychologist, they are implemented primarily at home by the parent. Most parents see significant improvement in their children's eating habits within three months.

If your infant is having problems with breast- or bottle-feeding, step 7 describes our pre-chaining program, which will help you develop your baby's feeding skills at the proper time and rate so he won't fall behind developmentally and develop feeding problems later on.

Step 8 will give you information and special strategies to help overcome your child's eating problems if he has autism, Down syndrome, or visual impairment.

DOES MY CHILD NEED A FEEDING TEAM?

You might be tempted to skip over the first five evaluation steps in the program and just start food chaining with your child—but we can't urge you strongly enough not to do this. Food chaining alone is unlikely to solve the issues your child has with eating. Whether your child is moderately finicky or has a serious feeding disorder, there may be many factors that contribute to his feeding problem, and the first five steps help you identify and resolve these factors so that food chaining can be successful. If your child's eating issues are significant enough for you to have picked up this book, we recommend that you play it safe and seek guidance from a feeding team.

HOW TO FIND A FEEDING TEAM FOR YOUR CHILD

There are some medical centers where an already assembled feeding team exists, but they may not be close enough to where you live to be feasible for you. There may also be a local feeding team in private practice or associated with your medical center with whom your pediatrician can put you in contact. If your pediatrician cannot refer you to a feeding team, ask him to refer you to a pediatric dietitian. Seeing a dietitian is the next step in the food-chaining process, helping you evaluate how much nutrition your child is getting and whether he may have food allergies, so you'll be on the right track.

If the pediatric dietitian cannot refer you to other members of a feeding team, you may need to assemble a team yourself. This may sound daunting, but it's actually not difficult. In each chapter of this book, we describe the type of medical professional your child may need for a particular step in the process and offer some advice on finding a professional in your area. You can always get referrals from your child's current doctors, ask your friends or your child's school for referrals, or call your local hospital for information. The Internet is an invaluable resource and can help you find a feeding team close to you (do a search for "pediatric feeding teams").

One of the greatest aspects of food chaining is that it can work in conjunction with other treatment approaches. You can take your child to be assessed by a feeding team hundreds of miles away, and they can work with your local health-care practitioners to implement food chaining. If you do have to put together your own feeding team, they can easily share information on your child by filling out one notebook that travels to each health-care practitioner with your child or by taping their sessions with your child so every team member can observe them. After your child has been fully assessed, the health-care practitioners can contribute the results of their evaluations to a comprehensive letter addressed to your child's pediatrician.

Having a local feeding team is certainly helpful but not necessary to food chaining. However, if you would feel more comfortable using the services of an established feeding team, regardless of their distance from your home, here are some guidelines for choosing the right one.

Does the team address your concerns? The members of a feeding team should properly identify themselves and their role in your child's feeding program. They should be good listeners and attend to your needs and your child's. Upon your child's initial evaluation, you should feel that an adequate care plan has been provided by experienced and empathetic care providers. Depending on your child's feeding disorder and deficiencies, consultation with specialists in speech therapy, occupational therapy, nutrition, oral head and neck surgery, general surgery, gastroenterology, and psychology should be readily available.

Are they providing attainable goals for your child? No two kids' eating problems are exactly alike, and each child should be evaluated and treated individually. A treatment plan should be based specifically upon your child's needs. A program should clearly define what the therapist will do versus your role and your child's role. Parents are not feeding therapists, and you should not be put in the overwhelming position of assuming that role. Instead, you should facilitate therapy as directed by feeding team members. Look for a team that values your feedback as to what's working and what's not—you know your child best.

Are they willing to work with your local physicians? Many feeding programs are located in urban or regional health centers that, depending on where you live, may not be convenient to get to on a regular basis. Therefore, feeding-team members should be willing and able to work closely with your local health-care providers, who can help execute your child's treatment plan. Follow-up with the feeding team may be required on occasion for reassessment.

Can you get in touch quickly if your child runs into a problem? The feeding process is dynamic and is influenced by many factors, from a bad day at school to the atmosphere at a birthday party. In order to meet and overcome these challenges on a day-to-day basis, frequent communication between you and your child's feeding team is essential. Immediate feedback through phone calls, e-mail, or even video is best. Feeding-team members should provide anticipatory feeding guidance for common problems that occur during therapy. They should be accessible to you and your child's other caretakers, including day cares and schools, and should be in contact with your child's primary care physician regarding their evaluation of your child and his treatment plan.

Good communication requires a great deal of patience. Misunderstandings are not uncommon, especially when you're dealing with several health-care practitioners at one time. Do not be afraid to ask questions if you need the team to clarify a diagnosis or a recommendation. Diagnosis can be a long process, so it's important to have a clear understanding of the team's philosophy and program.

Are they willing to take on the challenge? Depending on the severity of your child's condition, the treatment may be tedious. You need to feel confident your team is there to help alleviate any feelings of frustration and exhaustion this may cause. Your child's feeding team should be trustworthy and approachable and possess knowledge, empathy, and integrity. They should be committed for the long haul. The greatest reward for a good feeding team is seeing children overcome feeding challenges, no matter how long or how much work it takes.

YOUR CHILD *CAN* GET PAST THIS

Feeding disorders can be very difficult to cope with. It is frustrating and draining to deal with your child's tantrums and food refusals day after day, not to mention the constant worrying about whether your child is eating enough. We know this not just from a professional standpoint, but from a personal one as well. Cheri's son suffers from cyclic vomiting syndrome (see chapter 1 for more details on this condition and Cheri's story), and Sibyl's son has sensory issues that make it difficult for him to touch certain foods and gives him very strong food preferences. We know firsthand that the love you have for your child can make you desperate to get him to eat, and you may have tried many different tactics to accomplish that. Unfortunately, many times our strong parental instinct to fix our child's feeding problem combined with our lack of understanding about what is causing it can drive us to do the wrong thing for them, such as push too hard, be too strict or too lenient, or give our child gifts or money for eating. Each child's eating issue is unique and requires an individualized solution. For instance, if your child simply *can't* eat because of a medical problem or a sensory processing disorder, forcing him or her to try will only intensify the problem. You've probably picked up this book because you are at your wit's end and don't know where to turn next. We are very happy to tell you that studies have proven that the food-chaining program *can* help your child overcome his feeding problem—and this makes for happier mealtimes for the whole family. Dinner-table tension and fights will become a thing of the past, because the relationship between your family, your child, and food will become safe and positive. You have a lot to look forward to. Soon your child will be eating a better-balanced diet—and enjoying it!

CHAPTER 1

Could a Health Problem Be Causing My Child's Picky or Problem Eating?

The Medical Evaluation

Seven-year-old Sally is refusing to eat many of her meals, telling her mother, Megan, that she's not hungry. Sally has always been picky, but naturally her mother is worried. In addition, Sally has had a frequent cough for weeks now that doesn't seem to be getting any better, and she's been complaining at night that her chest burns. Last week she vomited after a meal, and it's happened two more times since then. Megan has done everything she can think of to help Sally feel better, from giving her over-the-counter medications to cooking her favorite foods, but nothing has worked. Megan has decided that it's time to take Sally to see her pediatrician and find out what's going on.

IT'S POSSIBLE THAT your child suffers from a medical condition that is causing or at least contributing to her eating issues. Gastroesophageal reflux disease (GERD), breathing problems, and severe constipation are just a few of the health conditions that can cause your child to refuse to eat or only want to eat certain foods. For instance, when Megan took Molly to the pediatrician's office, she learned that Molly was suffering from GERD, which was causing her persistent cough, heartburn, and vomiting. Inflammation of her **esophagus** (also called **esophagitis**) was making eating painful for Molly. As illustrated in this case, identifying or ruling out the presence of a medical condition in your child is an important first step in the food-chaining process. If a medical condition does exist, your child's eating problem cannot be tackled until the condition is either resolved or under control.

In this chapter, you will learn about the symptoms that indicate that your child may have a health condition, how to determine which condition might be affecting your child, and strategies for treating it. A vast majority of medical conditions associated with picky and problem eating involve either the upper airway or digestive tract. Here's a list of the common symptoms that indicate a health condition may be causing or contributing to your child's eating issues:

- Vomiting
- Retching while eating
- Choking
- Colic
- Spitting up
- Gagging on food
- Coughing
- Heartburn

- Diarrhea
- Difficult or painful swallowing
- Noisy breathing
- Wheezing
- Hives
- Constipation
- Food stuck in throat
- Pneumonia
- Rash
- Lack of appetite

The frequency, intensity, and duration of these symptoms vary from child to child. Over time, some symptoms may improve, worsen, or even overlap. As you can see, some symptoms, such as retching while eating or lack of appetite, have a clear relationship to eating difficulties, while others are less apparent. Most of the conditions we discuss in this chapter share many of the same symptoms (particularly the gastrointestinal conditions), so it's very important that you don't try to diagnose your child yourself. If you have any concerns about your child's eating habits, and especially if your child is currently showing one or more of these symptoms, she should be examined by her pediatrician.

GROWTH CHARTS

These growth charts are used by your child's pediatrician to determine whether she is growing and gaining weight properly. He will individually plot your child's weight, height, and head circumference according to her age. These charts also help the pediatrician determine whether your child's weight is proportional to her height. A different set of charts is used for older children.

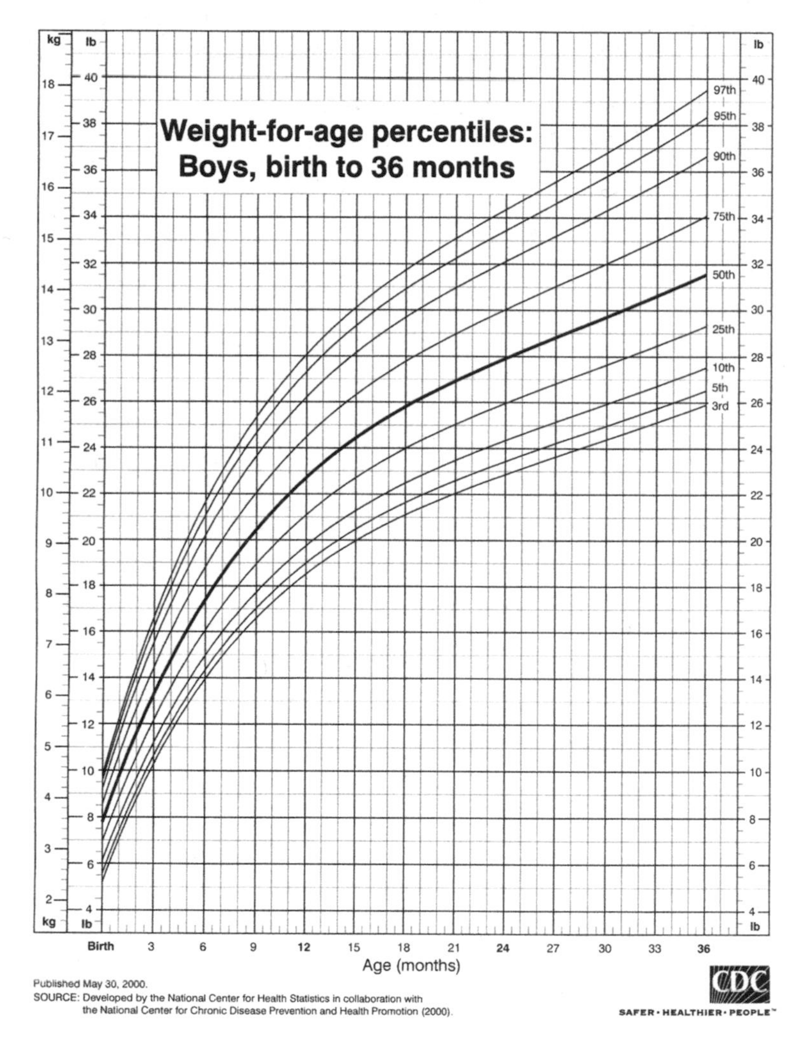
CDC Growth Charts: United States
Weight-for-age percentiles:
Boys, birth to 36 months
kg
lb
97th
95th
90th
75th
50th
25th
10th
5th
3rd
Birth
3
6
9
12
15
18
21
24
27
30
33
36
Age (months)
Published May 30, 2000.
SOURCE: Developed by the National Center for Health Statistics in collaboration with
the National Center for Chronic Disease Prevention and Health Promotion (2000).
CDC
SAFER · HEALTHIER · PEOPLE™

CDC Growth Charts: United States

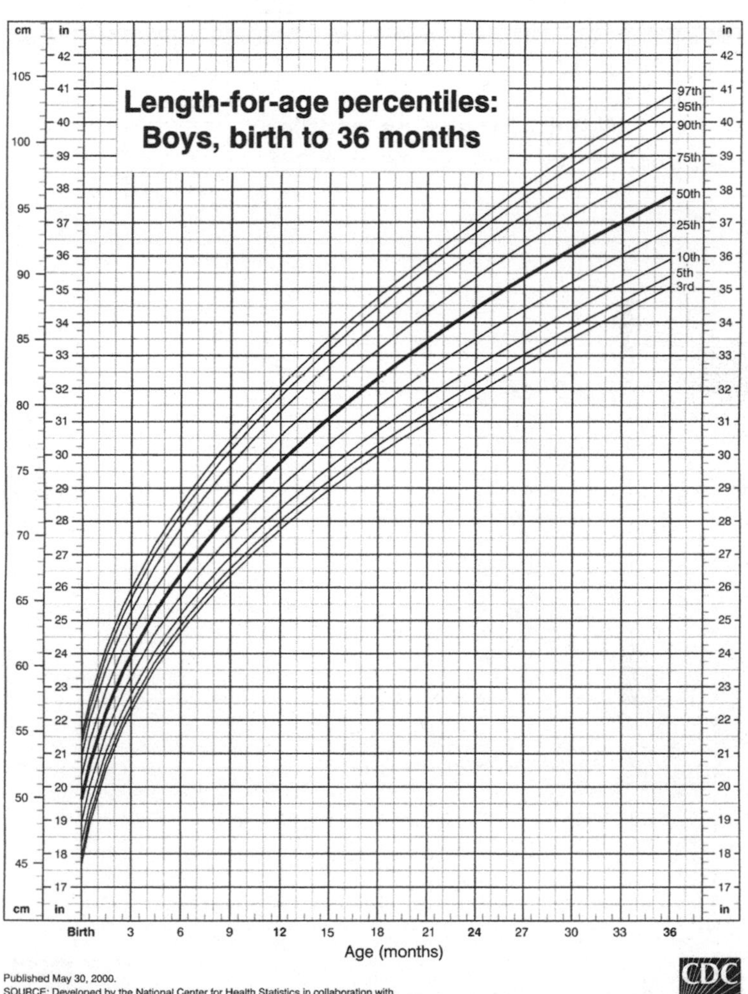

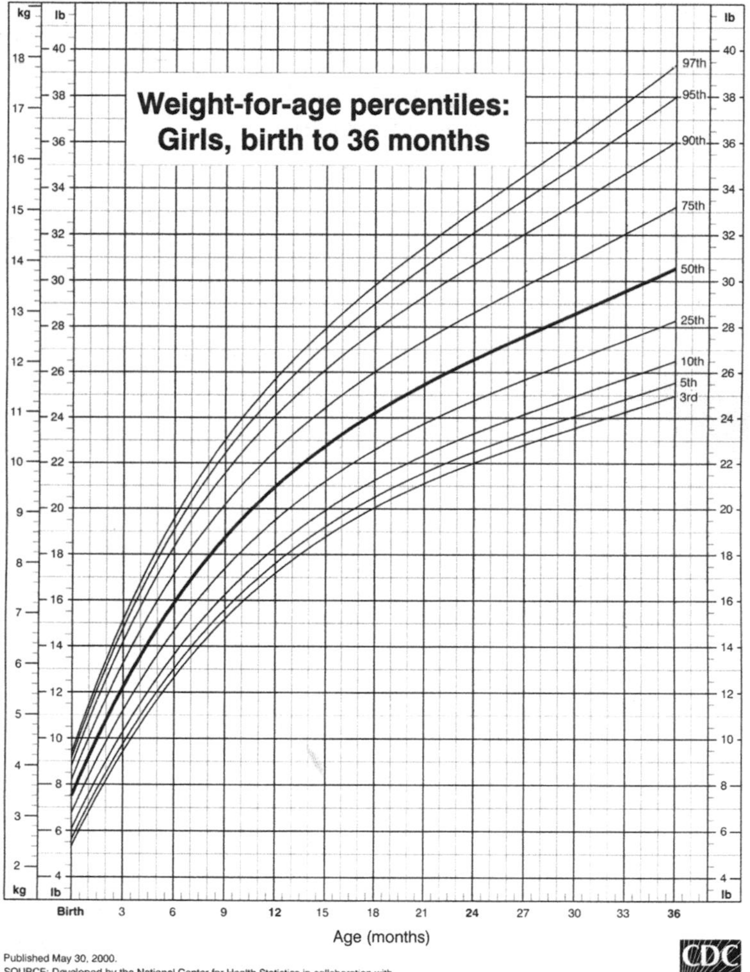
CDC Growth Charts: United States
Weight-for-age percentiles:
Girls, birth to 36 months
kg
lb
97th
95th
90th
75th
50th
25th
10th
5th
3rd
Birth
3
6
9
12
15
18
21
24
27
30
33
36
Age (months)
Published May 30, 2000.
SOURCE: Developed by the National Center for Health Statistics in collaboration with
the National Center for Chronic Disease Prevention and Health Promotion (2000).
CDC
SAFER · HEALTHIER · PEOPLE

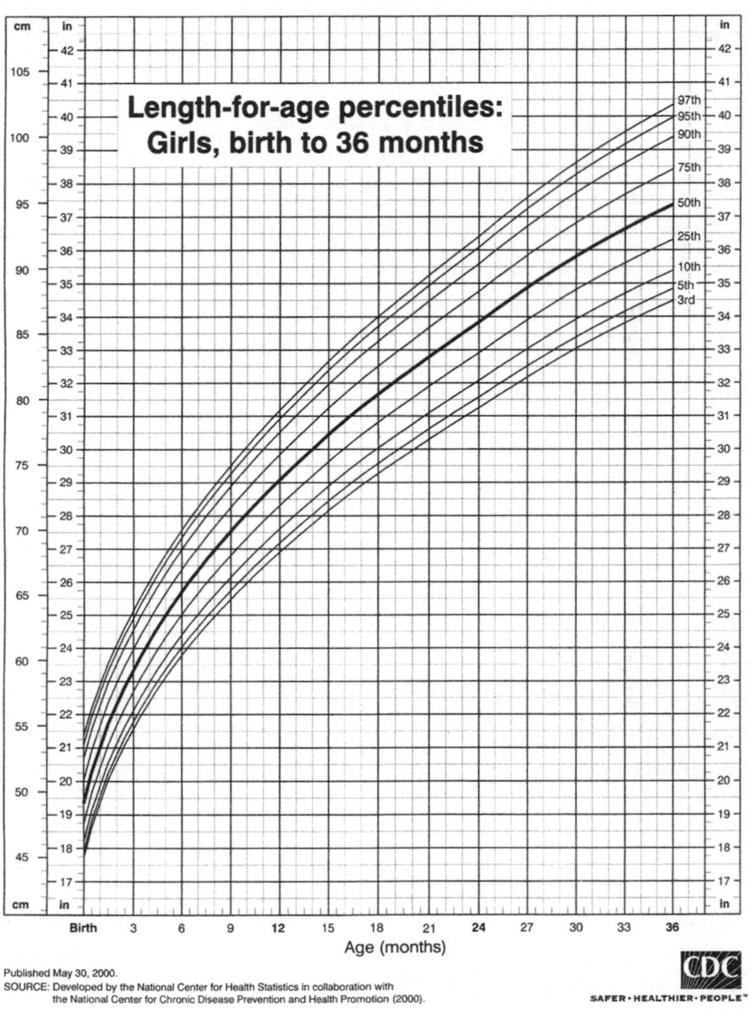
CDC Growth Charts: United States
Length-for-age percentiles:
Girls, birth to 36 months
cm
in
97th
95th
90th
75th
50th
25th
10th
5th
3rd
Birth
3
6
9
12
15
18
21
24
27
30
33
36
Age (months)
Published May 30, 2000.
SOURCE: Developed by the National Center for Health Statistics in collaboration with the National Center for Chronic Disease Prevention and Health Promotion (2000).
CDC
SAFER • HEALTHIER • PEOPLE

WHAT TO EXPECT AT THE PEDIATRICIAN EXAM

Visiting your child's pediatrician is the first step in identifying whether your child may have a health problem that is causing or contributing to her eating difficulties. The pediatrician will perform a basic medical evaluation on your child. This means he will do a routine physical exam and check for abnormalities, including small or large head size, heart murmur, decreased vigor, weak cry, enlarged liver or spleen, and wheezing. He will also assess her nutritional status by checking her weight, height, and head circumference (in infants). You may have noticed that the pediatrician notes your child's weight, height, and head circumference at every one of your visits. By plotting these parameters on a growth chart at regular intervals, he can detect any abnormalities in your child's rate of growth. The pediatrician may order noninvasive diagnostic testing on your child, such as blood, urine, or stool tests, to screen for disorders involving poor absorption of nutrients, infection, and chronic inflammation. He may also order X-ray studies to visualize disorders of the gastrointestinal (GI) or urinary tract. If the physical examination or the diagnostic testing points to a particular disorder, the pediatrician may request a consultation from a pediatric subspecialist trained to deal with that disorder.

BREATHING DIFFICULTIES

Sometimes children resist food because they can't properly breathe or swallow.

If your child has **stridor** (noisy breathing) or hoarseness, she may need to see an otolaryngologist (an eye, ear, nose, and throat doctor) who treats disorders of the upper airway. The oral head and neck physician will examine your child to make sure that her tonsils, adenoids, and vocal cords are not causing problems. If your child cannot breathe through her nose (which is necessary for bottle-feeding), she may have problems coordinating the suck/swallow/breathe sequence, which is a very important feeding skill (see chapter 4 for more information on this sequence). If her vocal cords don't close, the larynx won't elevate and pull itself out of the way for safe swallowing. Typically these problems require a change in how feedings are administered, medical treatment (such as nasal sprays or medications), or surgery to remove the tonsils and adenoids. More commonly, though, kids' feeding problems are caused by disorders of the GI tract.

GASTROINTESTINAL PROBLEMS

If the pediatrician suspects that your child has a GI disorder, your child may need to see a **pediatric gastroenterologist** for additional testing. Pediatric gastroenterologists are doctors specifically trained to evaluate and treat children with digestive disorders.

A gastroenterologist will also reassess your child's nutritional status to determine whether her nutritional needs are being met. If not, your child may require either supplemental tube feedings or intravenous solutions (see chapter 8 for more information on tube feedings). It's critically important that your child get the nutrition that she needs, so if she is malnourished, replenishing her nutrient levels will take top priority, and her feeding program may be put on hold until she is deemed healthy enough to continue.

If an evaluation indicates your child suffers from a digestive disorder, the gastroenterologist will devise a specific treatment plan, which will be implemented and supervised over a series of office visits. The contribution of the gastroenterologist to a feeding program is different for every child, but his role is crucial. GI problems must be identified and treated or they will prevent your child from overcoming her feeding disorder.

After the physician has examined your child for telltale signs and symptoms, he will likely have a good idea of which GI disorder your child may have. The next step is to administer tests to verify his tentative diagnosis. Based on your child's symptoms, she'll likely be tested for one or more of the following conditions.

GASTROESOPHAGEAL REFLUX (GER)

The most common symptoms are:

- Spitting up
- Vomiting
- Colicky behavior
- Persistent sore throat

When you swallow, food passes down your throat and through your esophagus to your stomach. At the bottom of the esophagus lie muscles that control the **lower esophageal sphincter,** the opening between the esophagus and the stomach. The lower esophageal sphincter normally remains tightly closed except when you swallow food. When this muscle opens at other times, the acid-containing contents of the stomach may travel back up into the esophagus. This backward flow is called gastroesophageal reflux (GER). Spitting up, vomiting, or regurgitation with GER is patternless, meaning it may occur at any time after a meal, several minutes to several hours later.

GER occurs in approximately 80 percent of infants. Children with GER spit up or even projectile-vomit frequently during infancy, particularly during the first six months. Some babies are "happy spitters"—in other words, their GER doesn't bother them and they gain weight well, feed well, and otherwise thrive. Other babies are not as fortunate and exhibit colicky behavior and feeding difficulties. The good news is that GER is considered a benign condition that doesn't lead to long-term problems, affect growth or development, or even require medical intervention. Most babies will outgrow the condition by their first birthday. It's important to note, however, that some infants outgrow GER and still have feeding difficulties.

GASTROESOPHAGEAL REFLUX DISEASE (GERD)

The most common symptoms are:

- Frequent or recurrent vomiting
- Frequent or persistent cough (nonseasonal)
- Choking or gagging while eating
- Heartburn, colicky behavior
- Regurgitation and reswallowing

Gastroesophageal reflux disease (GERD) is reflux that causes disease in the GI tract (i.e., esophagitis) or lungs (i.e., wheezing, **aspiration,** or pneumonia). Unlike GER, which affects only infants, GERD can affect children of any age.

DIAGNOSING GERD

If the pediatric gastroenterologist suspects your child has GERD, he will order one or more of the following tests to confirm his diagnosis, as well as to exclude the presence of other conditions:

- **Upper GI X-ray.** This is a special X-ray test performed by a **radiologist** that uses barium to highlight the esophagus, stomach, and upper part of the small intestine. This test may identify any obstructions or narrowing in these areas. An upper GI X-ray is usually performed in a hospital radiology department and will take less than an hour to complete. The test is not invasive and should not cause your child any discomfort.
- **Gastric-emptying study.** If your child vomits frequently a few hours after a meal, her stomach may be emptying too slowly. A gastric-emptying test is used to determine how rapidly the stomach empties. During a gastric-emptying test, your child drinks milk or eats food mixed with radio-labeled milk. Immediate and delayed images of the stomach and esophagus are obtained using a special

camera. The procedure is performed in a nuclear medicine suite at a hospital and takes approximately 90 minutes to complete. This test is noninvasive, does not expose your child to harmful radiation, and should not cause her any discomfort.

- **Upper GI endoscopy.** In this procedure, a gastroenterologist (or sometimes an **endoscopist**) will use an **endoscope,** or a thin, flexible, lighted tube and camera, to look directly inside your child's esophagus, stomach, and upper part of the small intestine, and take biopsies. The **biopsy** specimens are processed and examined under a microscope for abnormalities. An endoscopy is performed either at a hospital or an outpatient center equipped to handle children undergoing **sedation.** Sedatives or hypnotics are administered by an attending **anesthesiologist** or sometimes the gastoenterologist himself. Your child will recover from the procedure in about an hour and should experience no pain during or after the procedure. Endoscopy has minimal risks, but you should discuss them with the gastroenterologist before the procedure. Be sure to alert the anesthesiologist and gastroenterologist to any allergies your child has to medications so as to avoid any side effects from anesthetics they may use during the procedure.
- **pH probe.** Prolonged pH monitoring is performed to determine the presence and severity of acid reflux

> over an entire day and night. The test is often performed to determine the necessity of antireflux surgery or whether antireflux surgery has failed. To perform the study, a pH probe (a long, thin tube with an acid sensor at the tip) is passed through your child's nose, down the back of the throat, and into the lower portion of the esophagus, where it will be positioned for 24 hours. The study may be performed at home or in the hospital, and your child will be encouraged to go about her day as normally as possible during the test. Since a pH probe involves measuring acidity, your child will typically be asked not to take any acid-blocking medications for a few days prior to the test (see page 15 later in this chapter for more information on acid-blocking medications). The test tells the gastroenterologist how much acid reflux occurred and also connects reflux activity to particular "events," such as coughing, wheezing, or heartburn sensation.

Both the upper GI endoscopy and the pH probe are invasive tests and are usually performed only if a change in your child's medical treatment or surgery is being considered.

TREATMENT FOR GERD

If your child has reflux symptoms, these changes are often recommended:

- Position your infant upright, perhaps against your chest, for 20 minutes after each feeding.
- Avoid using an infant seat or swing for 20 minutes after each feeding.
- If you have an older child, make sure she avoids consuming caffeinated beverages or chocolates containing caffeine.
- Raise the head of your child's crib or bed so she's no longer lying flat.
- Try an over-the-counter gas-relief medication such as Mylicon or Gaviscon. For older children, try Mylanta or Maalox.

If none of these suggestions relieve your child's problem, the gastroenterologist may suggest a trial of these medications:

MEDICATIONS

Zantac or other histamine-2 receptor antagonists. Also known as H2-blockers, this class of drugs prevents or blocks the production of gastric acid. These medications are often used to relieve mild symptoms and are very safe. The most commonly prescribed H2-blockers are Zantac (ranitidine) and Tagamet (cimetidine). These medications are also available over the counter.

Prilosec or other proton pump inhibitors. Proton pump inhibitors, like H2-blockers, also reduce acid production in the stomach, but they are much more potent. They also have minimal side effects and are used to treat children of all ages. The most commonly prescribed proton pump inhibitors are Prevacid (lansoprazole) and Nexium (esomeprazole). Over-the-counter preparations are also available, including Prilosec (omeprazole).

Reglan (metoclopramide hydrochloride). This medication is used to hasten the movement of food through the stomach and intestines. However, Reglan is associated with some serious side effects involving the central nervous system, such as increased irritability and fussiness.

Erythromycin. A low dose of this antibiotic is used to enhance stomach emptying, a problem often associated with diabetes. It has been known to cause abdominal discomfort, so be sure to discuss this side effect with your child's doctor.

SURGERY

Children with severe, chronic GERD may need surgery to correct the problem, particularly if their symptoms are not relieved through medical treatment or they are experiencing a life-threatening complication such as aspirating food into their lungs. When surgery is necessary, **fundoplication** is the most commonly performed procedure. A fundoplication involves wrapping the upper curve of the stomach (the **fundus**) around the lower esophagus and sewing it into place so that the lower portion of the esophagus passes through a small tunnel of stomach muscle. This surgery strengthens the lower esophageal sphincter, or the valve between the esophagus and stomach, which stops acid from backing up into the esophagus easily.

Fundoplication is usually effective, but it is not without risk. Possible side effects include excess gas, bloating caused by gas buildup, retching, swallowing problems, and pain at the surgical site. These complications happen more often in children with disabilities such as cerebral palsy or severe developmental delay. Be sure to discuss the potential risks and benefits of this operation with your child's gastroenterologist.

DID YOU KNOW?

Dehydration, which is the excessive loss of fluid due to vomiting, diarrhea, or both, can be a dangerous, even life-threatening condition. If your child shows signs of dehydration such as dry mouth, absence of tears, sunken fontanel (soft spot on skull), and decreased urination, or is experiencing prolonged vomiting spells, contact your doctor immediately. She may need to be rehydrated orally with a rehydration fluid like Pedialyte or intravenously if she can't keep liquids down.

IDIOPATHIC EOSINOPHILIC ESOPHAGITIS (IEE)

The most common symptoms are:

- Coughing, gagging, or choking while feeding
- Vomiting
- Poor weight gain
- Food caught in esophagus
- Eczema
- Asthma
- Hives

Twenty-month-old Matthew had been gagging and aversive to food since nine months of age. He also had severe eczema from the age of three months. His parents switched him to soy formula and then to a hypoallergenic formula, but neither improved his eczema. Skin testing showed Matthew to be allergic to milk and eggs, so his parents removed milk, soy, and egg products from his diet and changed to rice milk. Still, his feeding aversion persisted, and his eczema did not improve.

Children who don't respond to antireflux medications or who have progressive symptoms such as coughing, gagging, or choking in association with feeding may not have GERD after all. Instead, they may have a condition called **idiopathic eosinophilic esophagitis (IEE),** which is an inflammation of the esophagus caused by an allergic-type response rather than an acid injury. IEE is diagnosed solely through endoscopy and biopsy, which is performed at either an endoscopist's office or a hospital.

IEE is not treated with acid-blocking medication like GERD, but rather with a restrictive diet and/or corticosteroid medication (given by mouth or inhaler). The restrictive diet excludes the foods that are most likely causing your child's problem, such as dairy products, soy, eggs, seafood, wheat, and peanuts, and then reintroduces them one or two at a time to test your child's tolerance. In an infant's case, she would be switched to a specialized low-allergy formula. Allergy testing such as a **patch test, skin prick,** or **RAST** (see chapter 2 for more information on allergies and allergy testing) is often used to help identify your child's food allergies, but the results are not always definitive. The restrictive diet (and specialized formula) has proven to be very successful for most children and appears to have a more lasting effect than corticosteroids. As with GER, your child's feeding problems may linger despite proper treatment for the condition.

Matthew underwent an upper endoscopy and was diagnosed with IEE. We put him on an elemental formula and diet for four weeks, at which time he was rescoped and we determined that his esophagus had healed. Since his diagnosis and treatment for IEE, Matthew's desire to eat has significantly increased, and he is currently accepting a wider variety of foods. His food-chaining program has been successful because we were able to identify and treat his underlying medical condition.

ACUTE PAINFUL SWALLOWING

The most common symptom is:

- Abrupt food refusal

Occasionally, a child with no previous history of GER or GERD may experience a sudden onset of painful swallowing. In these instances, an infection (typically viral) may be causing esophagitis, or the swelling of the esophagus. This diagnosis, like reflux and IEE, is established by an endoscopy. In otherwise healthy children, the condition should improve spontaneously over several days and require no medication.

However, if your child has a deficient or suppressed immune system caused by disease or chemotherapy, she may require specific antiviral or antifungal therapy.

MOTILITY-RELATED GI CONDITIONS

There are other GI disorders that affect feeding which involve **motility,** or the way that food moves through the esophagus, stomach, and intestines. Your child's gastroenterologist may test her for the following disorders as well:

Diarrhea

The most common symptoms are:

- Watery, liquid stool
- Abdominal cramps

Diarrhea is defined as loose, watery stool that may occur several times a day. There are several causes for diarrhea in children, but it's most commonly due to a viral infection. All children get acute diarrhea once in a while, which usually lasts for several days before getting better on its own. However, some kids suffer from severe bouts of diarrhea that put them at risk for dehydration and may be a sign of a more serious health problem. There is no specific treatment for viral-induced diarrhea. However, rehydration fluids (e.g., Pedialyte) are usually recommended during the course of the illness to prevent dehydration from occurring, especially for infants who are more susceptible to dehydration than older children and adults. Within a day or so, infant formula or breast-feeding should replace rehydration fluid, as it lacks sufficient calories and nutrients for prolonged use.

Constipation

The most common symptoms are:

- Hard, dry, small stools that are difficult to pass
- Large, infrequent bowel movements

Constipation is defined as having a bowel movement fewer than three times per week. It is a frequent occurrence in children, especially those on a restrictive diet or living with disabilities. A child's appetite and intake may be adversely affected by severe constipation, so aggressive treatment involving laxative therapy is usually recommended. The most commonly prescribed and effective laxatives are mineral oil, milk of magnesia, Kristalose (lactulose), Miralax, and Glycolax (both polyethylene glycol solutions). There are minimal side effects or risk factors associated with these laxatives, even if your child is using them for several weeks or even months.

Bowel obstruction

The most common symptoms are:

- bile-tinged (or greenish) vomit
- abdominal pain and cramping

A bowel obstruction is a blockage of the intestines that prevents the normal transit of the products of digestion. A bowel obstruction is generally diagnosed with X-rays of the abdomen. Surgical correction is usually required.

Chronic intestinal pseudo-obstruction (CIP)

The most common symptoms are:

- bile-tinged vomit
- abdominal pain and cramping

Chronic intestinal pseudo-obstruction is a rare disorder of GI motility in which coordinated contractions (**peristalsis**) in the intestinal tract become altered and insufficient. The symptoms of CIP are similar to those of a bowel obstruction, but there is no obstruction. CIP is diagnosed based on symptoms and findings after a physical examination, plus the proven absence of a true bowel obstruction. This condition tends to wax and wane over a lifetime and cannot be corrected with surgery. If your child has chronic intestinal pseudo-obstruction, she may require intravenous nutrition to meet her nutritional needs.

CYCLIC VOMITING SYNDROME (CVS)

The most common symptoms are:

- Sudden, rapid, frequent, and intense vomiting lasting hours to several days
- Abdominal pain
- Feeling of weakness
- Sweating or chills
- Fever
- Rapid heart rate
- Paleness

- Headache
- Strong thirst
- Sensitivity to light and noise
- Exhaustion
- Drowsiness
- Impaired concentration
- Irritability

Cyclic vomiting syndrome is not specifically a GI-related disorder, but there is some overlap, and we see enough children with the condition to warrant a section on it. CVS is a condition in which children experience episodes of overwhelmingly intense nausea and vomiting with or without abdominal pain. The vomiting is usually rapid and frequent and often requires a trip to the emergency room. Cyclic vomiting syndrome occurs suddenly, can last hours to several days, and then abruptly disappears, followed by symptom-free periods of weeks to months.

There is no known cause for CVS, though it is thought that the condition may overlap with other digestive disorders such as **delayed gastric emptying** (also known as **gastroparesis**) as well as diabetes. Children with cyclic vomiting can also have many feeding-related issues, such as esophagitis and discomfort with eating.

CVS AND MIGRAINE

Researchers believe that there is a connection between migraine and CVS, though the relationship is still unclear.

Both migraine headaches and CVS have severe symptoms that start quickly and end abruptly, followed by longer periods without pain or other symptoms. Research has also shown that many children with CVS either have a family history of migraine or develop migraines as they grow older. Because of the similarities between migraine and CVS, doctors treat some people with severe CVS with drugs that are also used for migraine headaches. The drugs are designed to prevent episodes, reduce their frequency, or lessen their severity.

SYMPTOMS

A CVS "attack" often begins with mild nausea, a lack of appetite, food refusal, feelings of weakness, an urgent feeling to move bowels, sweating or chills, and vague abdominal pain or pressure.

In the vomiting phase of an attack, your child may experience intense and frequent nausea and vomiting, paleness, exhaustion, drowsiness, impaired concentration, and irritability. Many kids experience a CVS attack when they are ill with another condition, such as strep throat or flu, and may also have a high fever, rapid heart rate, headache, severe abdominal pain, strong thirst, and sensitivity to noise and light.

As the attack passes, your child's appetite will gradually return and she will be able to keep food down. Her energy level will also return to normal as she becomes rehydrated. She will appear completely normal between attacks.

If your child suffers from CVS, she will need medical attention during her attacks. Early medical intervention is ideal, as it will decrease the duration of an episode.

DIAGNOSIS

Cyclic vomiting syndrome is hard to diagnose because no test exists to identify it. A doctor must diagnose CVS by looking at your child's symptoms and medical history and excluding more common diseases or disorders that can also cause nausea and vomiting, such as twisting of the bowel, **obstructive disorders,** and **mitochondrial disorders.** Also, diagnosis takes time, because doctors need to identify a pattern or cycle to the vomiting.

TREATMENT

There is no cure for cyclic vomiting syndrome, but there are ways to control some of the symptoms. Your child's doctor may prescribe medications to prevent a vomiting episode, stop or alleviate one that has already started, or relieve other symptoms, such as abdominal pain. Dehydration is a very real danger, especially for children, and severe nausea and vomiting may require hospitalization and intravenous fluids to prevent dehydration during an attack.

CHERI'S STORY

Identifying and diagnosing cyclic vomiting syndrome can be a difficult journey. I know this because my son Luke suffers from it. Luke started vomiting one day when he was eight months old. Although I felt the normal anxiety of being a new mom with a sick child, I assumed the vomiting would pass. But Luke didn't stop vomiting that day or the next, and it kept happening about every few minutes. I called the doctor and he gave me the usual medical advice about bowel rest (not giving Luke food or drink) and said that it would pass, but it didn't for two days. Luke lay in my lap and vomited night and day into a bowl and my husband would empty it and run back to us. I had never seen vomiting like this. I had no idea at that time that at that point, my child's life was threatened by dehydration.

These spells kept happening every 6 to 12 weeks and we got used to days of prolonged vomiting. We were terrified. When Luke turned two, he began to know when an episode was starting, and he would tell me, "Mommy, the monster is coming." And it was. I felt the monster, too. Luke was hospitalized many times for dehydration, or we would start out with an illness, such as strep throat or a virus, and move into a vomiting attack. This pattern would occur again and again for the next six years. In our years of searching for what was wrong with Luke, my husband, Randy, and I felt the pain only a parent knows, when you can't get anyone to listen to you and in your heart you know you haven't found the answers yet.

Enter the white knight . . . Luke's *third* pediatrician referred us to a pediatric GI specialist named Mark Fishbein. Randy and I went to what we thought would be just one more useless physician appointment. But

Dr. Fishbein came in, sat down with us, and acted like he had all the time in the world to listen. He asked me some of the same questions other doctors had asked, but he did it differently. I could tell he was *hearing* me. Then he said the words that changed our lives: *I think I know what is wrong with your son*. Luke had cyclic vomiting syndrome.

Dr. Fishbein set up a treatment plan for Luke that fought the monster and won, though CVS never completely goes away. Luke is 13 now, and we estimate that he has vomited 65,000 times in his life. We have lived through reflux, esophagitis, esophageal tears, no weight gain in a year, pain while eating, and a preference for drinking over eating, and I have seen my child suffer in ways that break my heart. If you are the parent of a child with CVS, or any GI disorder that affects eating, know that I've been where you are now. The best advice I can give you is never stop searching for a diagnosis and the right treatment for your child's medical problems. It's not always easy, but the answers are out there, so keep pushing.

We believe that children refuse to eat for a reason, and a legitimate medical condition may be affecting your child's desire or ability to eat. Now that you have either ruled out this possibility or discovered a health problem and taken steps to address it, your child has a far better chance of overcoming her picky or problem eating. In the next chapter, you'll learn how to ensure that your child is getting the nutrition she needs, and how to recognize and manage food allergies.

CHAPTER 2

Is My Child Getting Adequate Nutrition? Does She Have Food Allergies?

The Nutritional Evaluation

Nancy is worried about her eight-year-old son Brent. On the outside, he looks like a normal kid—he's gaining weight well, he has lots of energy, and he seems healthy. But over the last five years, Brent has gradually stopped eating most of the foods Nancy offers him. He refuses not only fruits and vegetables but meat as well, and the number of foods he accepts is continuing to decrease. Nancy has resorted to feeding him "junk food" all the time just so he'll eat something.

Brent's doctor told her repeatedly that he was just picky and would grow out of it, but the extent of the problem really hit home for Nancy when other family members started commenting about how he wouldn't eat anything. Nancy went to see the dietitian to find out what kind of vitamin she could give Brent so he could still be healthy even though he ate mostly junk food. There she discovered that many other people have children with similar feeding problems and that there was a way to improve her son's diet, his nutrition, and his overall health.

ONE OF THE main worries that many parents of picky and problem eaters have is whether their child is getting enough nutrition. The truth is that the narrower your child's diet, the more likely it is that he is missing some essential nutrients. If your child is unable to eat textured and/or table foods by 12 to 15 months of age, is not gaining adequate weight, or shows any of the other symptoms listed below, he has a feeding problem that should be evaluated by a pediatric dietitian.

In this chapter, you will learn what to expect at your appointment with the dietitian so you can arrive prepared to provide the information she will need from you. It's very important that you develop a solid understanding of your child's specific nutritional needs at every age so you can ensure that he meets them, so we offer guidelines on what and how much to feed your child from infancy through childhood and the teen years. This information will also help you determine if your child is experiencing problems with growth or eating, or is at risk for nutrient deficiencies. Finally, you will learn the facts about food allergies, which will help you determine if one or more allergies may be contributing to your child's eating problem.

SIGNS YOUR CHILD MAY NOT BE GETTING ENOUGH NUTRITION

When your child is not getting adequate nutrients for his body to perform properly, he is in danger of malnutrition. Malnutrition can be caused by an inadequate or unbalanced diet, digestive or malabsorption problems, or a medical condition such as **dysphagia**. It can be mild, with your child not showing any symptoms, or it can be severe, causing mental or physical disabilities, illness, and even death. Symptoms of malnutrition include:

- fatigue
- low energy
- dizziness
- irritability
- poor growth
- underweight
- weight loss
- dry skin
- poor immune function
- painful joints
- hair loss
- brittle nails
- loss of appetite
- shortness of stature compared to other children their age

In developed countries such as the United States, severe

malnutrition is rare. Children in developed countries are more apt to suffer from mild malnutrition, where they aren't getting enough of a specific nutrient, such as iron or calcium.

SIGNS YOUR CHILD MAY HAVE FOOD ALLERGIES

Food allergies are a big problem for many children today. In fact, studies show that the number of children suffering from food allergies has skyrocketed in the last three decades. Your child may have an allergy if he shows any of the following symptoms after eating:

- Hives, rash, eczema, itching
- Swelling of lips, face, tongue, or throat
- Sneezing, runny nose, nasal congestion, wheezing
- Abdominal pain, diarrhea, vomiting
- **Anaphylaxis** (a severe reaction that can result in constriction of the airways making it difficult to breathe, rapid pulse, and possible loss of consciousness)

Starting on page 64, we offer in-depth information on recognizing, diagnosing, and living with food allergies.

THE PEDIATRIC DIETITIAN APPOINTMENT

At this point, your child has been evaluated by his pediatrician (as well as the necessary pediatric subspecialists), and any underlying medical conditions that may be causing or contributing to his feeding problem have been either diagnosed or ruled out. The next step in the food-chaining program is to see a pediatric dietitian.

A pediatric dietitian is responsible for providing your child with overall nutritional care during the food-chaining program. She will perform a complete nutritional and growth assessment on your child, assess him for food allergies, evaluate his food and liquid intake before and during the process, conduct weekly weigh-ins, and select formula or caloric supplements for your child based on his unique needs. A pediatric dietitian will also manage tube feedings if they become necessary and provide nutritional treatment for your child if she has poor weight gain and failure to thrive.

Here's some advice for choosing the right pediatric dietitian for your child:

- Make sure you choose a registered dietitian (RD) and not just a nutritionist.
- If you can't find a pediatric dietitian in your area, make sure the dietitian you choose has experience working with children. Assessing nutritional status and creating care plans for children is much different than it is for adults.
- You can also contact the American Dietetic Association at www.eatright.org and (800) 877-1600 for a list of registered dietitians in your area.

At your initial visit, the pediatric dietitian will begin by asking you about your child's medical history, feeding history, and growth history. Here is a list of questions you will likely be asked:

- What was your child's birth weight and length?
- What was his gestational age? (Was he born at full term or preterm?)
- Has your child ever been hospitalized? What for?
- What (if any) medical diagnoses has your child been given by his pediatrician or other doctors?
- Is your child currently taking any medications?
- Does your child spit up or vomit? If so, how often and how much?
- Has your child been diagnosed with reflux? If so, is he taking medication for this problem?
- Does your child have constipation or diarrhea?
- Have you or your doctor ever been worried about your child's growth or weight gain?
- Does your child have any food allergies that you know of?
- Was your child breast-fed or bottle-fed? Did you have any difficulties with this?
- At what age did you begin to offer baby foods? Did you have any difficulties with this transition?
- At what age did you begin to offer table foods? Did you have any difficulties with this transition?
- Does your child have a feeding tube? If so, when was the feeding tube placed? What type of feedings does he receive and what type of formula?

Your answers to these questions will help the dietitian determine if there are any nutritional red flags in your child's medical history. For example, a child who has chronic diarrhea may not be absorbing all of the nutrients contained within the food he eats. The dietitian may ask further questions about the severity of your child's symptoms, when they occur, and if they relate to food. (This may lead her to refer your child to other specialists, such as a gastroenterologist.) Some medications can affect how certain nutrients are absorbed within your child's system, so if your child is taking a medication, the dietitian will want to make sure his diet includes plenty of foods that provide the nutrients he may be lacking.

HELPFUL HINT

An easy way to provide the dietitian with much of the information she needs is to ask your pediatrician to send your child's medical records to her office. Alternatively, you could have a copy of your child's records made and bring them with you to your initial visit.

The dietitian will measure your child's weight, height (or length for infants), and head circumference and compare this to his growth records. She may even create her own growth chart for your child with more detailed information than your pediatrician used. This is how the dietitian will assess whether your child is growing appropriately. She will also evaluate any laboratory work or other testing that was performed on your child by the pediatrician or pediatric subspecialists we discussed in chapter 1.

Next, a thorough history of your child's diet will be taken.

The pediatric dietitian will likely ask some or all of the following questions:

- What does your child drink (breast milk, formula, milk, juice, soda, tea, and so forth) and how much of these liquids does he drink in a day?
- If your baby is taking formula, how is it prepared?
- If your baby is taking formula, is it thickened with anything, such as cereal?
- Does your child eat strained or pureed baby foods or table foods?
- What is a typical breakfast, lunch, snack, and dinner for your child?
- Does your child eat fruits and vegetables?
- Does your child eat cheese, yogurt, or other dairy products?
- Does your child eat meat, fish, eggs, beans, or peanut butter?
- Does your child eat bread, cereal, pasta, or rice?
- Does your child receive any supplements, such as PediaSure?

In order to give the dietitian as complete and accurate a diet history as possible and help answer the above questions, we suggest you keep a food log for three to five days prior to your visit. A food log will also help the dietitian determine whether your child has any nutrient deficiencies or excesses, and it will help her to evaluate your child's meal and snack schedules.

Food Log

We suggest you create a food log and bring it to your first pediatric dietitian appointment. It will be a great help to your dietitian as she assesses your child and creates a customized nutrition care plan for him. Below is a sample food log to give you an idea of what yours should look like.

Child's name:_______________

Child's date of birth:_________

Instructions for completing the food log:

1. Try to record what your child has eaten or drunk immediately after the meal or snack so that the record is as accurate as possible.
2. Include at least two weekdays and one weekend day in your record. These should be consecutive days.
3. Include your child's name, date of birth, day of the week, and date on each page.
4. List each food on a separate line.
5. Specify amounts in terms such as teaspoons, tablespoons, cups, ½ slice, and dimensions of a piece of pizza or a serving of lasagna or meat. Terms like "a glassful" or "a bowlful" are not an accurate enough account of food consumed.
6. Don't forget about condiments (mayonnaise, butter, sugar).
7. Whenever possible, state the brand name, type of milk (skim, 2 percent, whole), and whether the food was fresh, frozen, or canned. Providing the list of ingredients in mixed dishes (like potato salad or lasagna) is also helpful.
8. Be sure to include everything, even liquids and candy.

Meal/Snack	Time of Day	Amount Consumed	Comments
Breakfast	7:30	¼ cup Cheerios 1 cup baby oatmeal mixed with 3 Tbsp pureed peaches 6 ounces apple juice	
Lunch	11:00	8 ounces Dannon yogurt 2 Tbsp SpaghettiOs with Parmesan cheese 4 ounces water	
Snack	2:00	7 ounces whole milk 8 animal crackers	
Dinner	5:30	5 ounces whole milk ½ cup mashed potatoes ½ cup peaches 3 bites turkey	
Bedtime Snack	8:00	½ cup popcorn 3 ounces orange juice	

Next, the dietitian will ask about your child's feeding skills, his mealtime environment, and his behaviors. Here are some of the questions you can expect her to ask:

- Does your child take a bottle? If so, what kind, and what is provided in the bottle?
- Does your child use a bottle, cup, spoon, or fork, or does he finger feed?
- Does your child feed himself?
- How often does your child eat (every ____hours, number of times per day, number of meals, number of snacks)?
- Does your child consume liquids with meals and snacks or throughout the day?
- How long do breast-/bottle-feedings, meals, or snacks take to complete?
- How do you know your child is hungry?
- How do you know your child is full or finished with a meal?
- What types of foods are easiest for your child to eat?
- What types of foods are most difficult for your child to eat?
- What position is your child in during feedings? (Is he in your lap, infant seat, flat on his back, in a high chair, regular chair, or booster seat?)
- Does your child have problems with gagging, choking, chewing, or swallowing foods?

This part of the assessment helps the dietitian determine if your child has a feeding problem and needs to see an occupational therapist or speech therapist for further evaluation. For example, say a two-year-old child drinks excessive amounts of milk and juice, and prefers only a few kinds of smooth and crunchy foods, while avoiding all other foods. He may have an oral motor skills problem or sensory problem that requires an evaluation and treatment from one or both of these therapists. Your answers to these questions will also help the dietitian understand which textures and flavors your child prefers. Then, the dietitian can use foods within these flavor and texture families (foods that your child is likely to eat because they are similar to the ones he already likes) to help make sure your child gets adequate nutrition.

After evaluating your child's medical, diet, and feeding history, the dietitian will decide if he needs vitamin and mineral supplements. If you are already giving him vitamin and mineral supplements, she will make sure they are appropriate for him. If your child is currently using a feeding tube, the dietitian will make sure that the tube feeding product and type of feedings he receives continues to be suitable.

Once the pediatric dietitian has assimilated all of the information she gathered at this initial appointment, she will create and implement a nutrition-care plan specially suited to your child's needs.

NUTRITIONAL GUIDELINES

"I want my child to eat his fruits and vegetables because I know they're good for him, but when I try to make him eat them, he either cries uncontrollably or they cause him to gag," says Shelley, mother of three-year-old Peter. Many parents assume that feeding their children a well-rounded diet should be easy, but that's simply not the case, especially for those of us raising picky or problem eaters. Establishing a nourishing diet for your child requires guidance, effort, and patience, and it begins the moment he is born. The next section of this chapter provides nutritional guidelines and advice for children of all ages, but particularly infants and toddlers. *Don't worry if your child is not meeting all of these standards*—the reality is that few children do. We offer these guidelines for two reasons: as standards to strive for and as benchmarks against which to measure your child's feeding problems. It's also important to keep in mind that your child is working through his feeding disorder and will not be a picky or problem eater forever. These guidelines can help you establish goals for your child when he reaches the food-chaining stage (see chapter 6).

INFANTS

Medical experts highly recommend that, when possible, you breast-feed your baby for the first year of his life. Breast-feeding is beneficial for many reasons. Studies have shown that it can protect babies from bacterial meningitis, ear infections, allergies, diarrhea, and respiratory tract infections. It may also decrease their risk for **sudden infant death syndrome (SIDS).** In older children and adults who were breast-fed, studies show a decreased incidence of some types of cancers, diabetes, asthma, obesity, and high cholesterol.

There are also many benefits for the breast-feeding mother. Women who breast-feed lose their pregnancy weight faster and are at reduced risk for developing breast and ovarian cancers and osteoporosis.

That said, breast-feeding is not always easy—or even possible for many women. Women who struggle with breast-feeding often feel like failures because they believe it should be a "natural" process that all mothers automatically know how to do. This is simply not the case. "When my baby had trouble breast-feeding and always seemed to cry when it was time to feed her, I felt like she was rejecting me and that I couldn't provide what she needed. I didn't know who to ask for help and I felt like my baby would be better off taking a bottle," said Jill, mom to two-year-old Lisa. The truth is that for many mothers and their infants, breast-feeding takes work as well as help from a professional, such as a **lactation consultant.** It's not uncommon for babies to develop feeding problems very early in life, and often a baby's difficulty with breast-feeding can indicate such a feeding problem. Don't be afraid to ask for help if you are having trouble breast-feeding or feel that things are just not as they should be (see the Resources section for information on the La Leche League).

HOW TO MEASURE YOUR SUCCESS AT BREAST-FEEDING

There are several simple indicators that can help you figure out whether your baby is breast-feeding successfully:

1. **Breast-feeding should not hurt.** If you're finding it painful, your baby may be having a problem latching on to your nipple properly. A proper latch

is important because it enables your baby to get an adequate amount of milk and it improves his oral motor skills. Pain during breast-feeding could also indicate engorgement or an infection called **mastitis.** If the pain doesn't subside after a day or two, you develop a fever or flu-like symptoms, or you suspect an infection, call your pediatrician or obstetrician for advice.

2. **You should be nursing often.** Newborns need to nurse 8 to 12 times in a 24-hour period for at least the first month of life. If you are breast-feeding less than this, your baby may not be getting an adequate amount of nourishment. Frequent nursing is also what keeps your milk supply high. It's all about supply and demand. A woman's body is designed to produce milk when the demand for it is there. Therefore, the more you breast-feed (or pump), the more milk you will produce. Alternatively, if you go for long periods (more than four hours) without nursing, your milk supply will decrease. After the first six to eight weeks, the number of times you nurse each day will decrease because your baby will begin to sleep for longer periods during the night and you will introduce solid foods to her diet at four to six months of age. Keep in mind that when your baby is going through a growth spurt, he may demand to nurse more often, which will again increase your milk supply.

3. **You can hear your baby swallowing.** Hearing your baby swallow during a nursing session is a sure sign that he is taking in your milk. Sometimes it's difficult for moms to tell whether their babies are swallowing, so ask another person to listen while you're nursing and tell you if they can hear it.
4. **Your baby's weight steadily increases.** It's common for new moms to be nervous about breast-feeding and worry their children won't get enough milk. The best way to determine whether your child is getting enough nourishment when you're breast-feeding is to have her weighed. Make an appointment to visit your pediatrician three to five days after leaving the hospital to have your baby weighed. Your baby should visit the pediatrician again at two to three weeks of age for another weight check. If your baby is gaining adequate weight, then you know she is receiving enough milk.

   On the other hand, if your baby is not gaining weight at the appropriate speed or she is losing weight, she may have a medical condition or a feeding problem. Your pediatrician will need to run tests and possibly consult with other specialists, such as a lactation consultant or a speech pathologist, to determine the reason for her poor weight gain. It's important to find out why your baby is not gaining weight well before turning to formula as a supplement to or a replacement for breast-feeding in order to prevent the feeding problem from recurring when you transition him back to all breast-feeding or to baby foods.

DID YOU KNOW?

Here are some interesting facts about nutrition and babies you may not be aware of:

- Infants don't need extra fluids, like water, until six months of age. Breast milk or formula provides them with an adequate amount of fluid. Water offers no nutrition and may fill your baby up, which can reduce his hunger and deprive him of the nutrition he needs from breast milk or formula.
- Feeding young infants cereal will not make them sleep longer at night.
- You can breast-feed even if your baby has a milk allergy.
- Your infant will experience the flavors of foods you eat because they are transferred through your breast milk.

BOTTLE-FEEDING

When breast-feeding doesn't work or is not possible, feeding your baby infant formula is a healthful option. Although formula does not contain some of the protective benefits that breast milk does, it does provide the nutrition your baby needs for the first year of his life. The most common infant formulas are cow's-milk-based, and that's likely what your pediatrician will recommend you feed your baby.

If you are bottle-feeding your baby and he exhibits signs of a feeding problem or fussiness around mealtimes, your first instinct will probably be to switch him to a new formula. Unfortunately, most feeding problems and fussiness are not resolved with numerous formula changes. Most of the families we have worked with tell us that changing from cow's milk to soy formula or a hypoallergenic formula did not solve their child's problem. That said, it's certainly worthwhile to try one formula change to see if the formula is indeed the problem. Keep in mind that infants need three or more days to get used to a change in formula, so don't expect immediate results. If a week has gone by and you see no improvement in your child's feeding problem, it's safe to assume the formula is not the culprit. Instead of buying an even more expensive special formula, call your pediatrician and explain that you tried a formula change, which made no difference, and you'd like to bring your baby in for further evaluation.

HOW MUCH SHOULD YOUR BABY BE EATING?

Below we've listed the guidelines that the medical community uses to guide infant feeding. It's important to note that these are just guidelines, and not every child will fit into these parameters. Perfectly healthy children have been known to consume both less and more of the amounts we list below. The best way to judge whether your baby has had enough to eat is to read her cues. Typical cues that your baby is full are: falling asleep during a feeding (after he has drunk a discernible amount of milk); turning away or becoming fussy after consuming some amount of food; and playing with the bottle. (See appendix 2, Feeding Your Baby and Young Child, for a complete set of guidelines.)

Age	Amount of Formula per Feeding	# of Feedings	Formula per Day
0–3 months	2–4 ounces	8–12	16–24 ounces
3–6 months	4–8 ounces	6–8	20–32 ounces
6–9 months	6–9 ounces	5–6	24–32 ounces
9–12 months	6–9 ounces	4–6	24–32 ounces

WHAT FORMULA SHOULD YOU USE?

There are several different formulas to choose from. Your pediatrician will likely recommend a particular type to use, or your obstetrician or the hospital staff where you give birth may suggest one, but it's good to know your options.

Cow's Milk. Cow's-milk-based formulas contain cow's milk protein and are the most common type of formula. Popular brands include Similac, Enfamil, and Carnation Good Start.

Soy. Soy-based formulas contain soy protein but may not be recommended for babies with a milk allergy, as they are also likely to be allergic to soy. Soy is lactose free and may be appropriate if your baby needs to avoid lactose. Popular brands include Isomil, ProSobee, and Carnation.

Hypoallergenic. Hypoallergenic formulas are partially digested and are designed for babies who have (or are suspected to have) a milk allergy. Some parents and pediatricians will use hypoallergenic formulas to see if it will soothe colic, but there is no research that proves that it relieves colic symptoms. If your baby is on a hypoallergenic formula and continues to have symptoms of a milk allergy, you should talk with your pediatrician about further testing. Popular brands are Nutramigen and Alimentum.

Enfamil A.R. This formula is designed specifically for infants with acid reflux (see chapter 1 for more information on GER and GERD). Enfamil A.R. contains rice starch, which thickens in the stomach when it combines with the stomach acid. This allows your baby to take the formula in its intended liquid form, but then thickens in the stomach to help limit reflux. However, if your baby is receiving medication for reflux, such as Prevacid, Prilosec, or Zantac, this formula may not be as effective in helping with reflux because it needs an acidic environment in order to thicken, and reflux medications are designed to reduce the acidic environment of the stomach. (Note: Under no circumstances should you thicken Enfamil A.R. with cereal. If your baby needs her formula thickened to promote safe swallowing, choose a different formula.)

DID YOU KNOW?

Sometimes it takes newborns a while to latch on to the nipple or coordinate the suck/swallow/breathe sequence while eating. These problems are normal and should resolve themselves within the first few weeks of life. Problem feeders, on the other hand, may consistently reject the breast or bottle, eat only while sleeping, or have lengthy feedings (more than 30 minutes).

MOVING ON TO SOLIDS

Most experts believe that babies should begin eating solid foods at between four and six months of age. Many recommend that you wait closer to six months, especially if you are breast-feeding, because your milk supply may decrease due to diminished demand from your baby. In fact, many babies are not developmentally ready to eat solid foods until closer to six months of age. Their digestive systems are still maturing and aren't equipped to handle solids foods until at least four months of age. Infants also have what's called the "extrusion reflex"—when you touch their tongue, they react by pushing their tongue forward. You may already be familiar with this—every time you put a spoonful of food in your baby's mouth, he pushes it right back at you with his tongue. It's not that your baby doesn't want the food; he just hasn't learned to control his extrusion reflex yet. At five or six months of age, your baby will begin opening his mouth in anticipation when he sees the spoon.

Here are some signs that your baby is ready to begin eating solid foods:

- **Good head control.** Your baby must be able to hold up his head when in a sitting position.
- **Can sit with support.** Your baby doesn't have to be able to sit unassisted but should be able to sit in a high chair without slumping or leaning to one side. You may want to position blankets or towels to help your baby maintain a good seated position. This

will make swallowing easier for him and help prevent choking.

- **Your baby shows interest in foods.** Often babies will lean forward, open their mouths in anticipation of a bite, or reach for food that you are eating.
- **Your baby has learned to control his tongue protrusion reflex.** The tongue protrusion reflex is present until age four to six months. The reflex protects your baby from choking by expelling any solid that enters his mouth. If your baby consistently pushes solid food out of his mouth with his tongue, wait a few days or a week and try again. You should never force food into your baby's mouth.

DID YOU KNOW?

You should not offer your baby solid foods in his bottle. Cereal mixed with formula to thicken it and prevent reflux has not been shown to be effective. (However, there are medical situations where thickening formula is required, such as if your baby is at risk for aspiration.) In order to teach feeding skills properly, you must offer your baby solid food by spoon. If your baby only takes solids from a bottle, this can delay the development of his feeding skills and put him at risk for choking.

Starting your baby on solid foods by six months of age is important because it teaches him the eating skills he will need to move on to more adult table foods. Breast milk or infant formula still provide all of your baby's nutritional needs at this stage, but baby food exposes him to new tastes and textures. You are not replacing breast milk or formula with baby food; you are simply adding a new element to your baby's diet. Your pediatrician will likely direct you to feed your baby only one (or even half of one) jar of stage I baby food a day for a while. Babies who are fed too much baby food may not drink enough breast milk or formula, which could lead to poor growth.

Be sure to start with single-ingredient foods so you can monitor your baby for food sensitivities. For example, if you're starting with fruits, you should offer your baby a particular fruit for three days in a row and watch him closely for any reaction to it. If he gets a rash or has vomiting or diarrhea, this may indicate he is allergic to that fruit. You should call your pediatrician to be sure. (More information on food allergies follows in this chapter.)

You will work your way through fruits, vegetable, meats, and cereals in this manner, until you're confident your baby has no food allergies (or his food allergies have been addressed). Then you can start offering him different foods mixed together, like turkey and peas or banana and raspberries.

DID YOU KNOW?

The order in which you introduce foods does not matter. A baby who receives fruits before vegetables will not dislike his vegetables when he gets older.

KEEP TRYING!

Exposure to new foods is critical for babies, and we urge you not to give up on new foods too fast. Don't assume that your baby will not eat a food just because he has rejected it a few times. It can take many tries before a baby will try something new, and he may decide he likes a food months or even years down the road. For example, many children who disliked baby-food peas when they were babies find they enjoy the table-food variety.

Portion sizes are very small at this stage—usually only a teaspoon to a tablespoon per meal—but it depends on the baby. Remember that your baby's appetite will vary from day to day. This means you'll need to adjust his portion size based on how he is accepting a particular meal in order to prevent over- or underfeeding. (See appendix 2, Feeding Your Baby and Young Child, for more detailed information.)

MAKING YOUR OWN BABY FOOD

Many parents wonder whether they should make their own baby food when the time comes to start their babies on solids. If you have the time and the inclination, making homemade baby food is a great idea. It costs less to make your own food than it does to buy it, and you can expose your baby to flavors you may not be able to find in commercially made products. For instance, you can offer exotic fruits such as pureed mango or papaya. Here are some guidelines for preparing homemade baby food:

1. Always wash your hands and clean the prep area well to prevent contamination.
2. Wash all produce well and remove peels and skins. Vegetables should be boiled or steamed prior to pureeing. We recommend you steam them—the vegetables will retain more of their nutrients. Here's a quick and easy cooking tip: steam them in the microwave for a fast meal.
3. Puree meats in the broth you used to cook the meat to keep the flavor.
4. Freeze extra food in ice cube containers or in small plastic containers for later use.
5. Be sure to label and date anything you freeze. You can safely freeze baby food for up to three months. Never refreeze baby food after it has thawed. Homemade baby food can be refrigerated for up to three days.
6. As long as you avoid the major allergens (wheat, soy, milk, eggs, fish, nuts, and peanuts) or have determined that your baby is not allergic to any of them (see page 67), anything you prepare for your family can be pureed for your baby. This way, you can prepare one meal for everyone and your baby can be part of your family mealtimes.

ADDING FLAVOR

In the United States, we tend to feed our babies very bland foods, but the truth is babies enjoy flavor just as much as we do.

In fact, your baby has already been exposed to myriad flavors through the foods you ate while he was in utero. If you breast-fed or are currently breast-feeding, your baby is being exposed through your breast milk to the flavors of everything you're eating. Many ethnic cultures expose their infants and toddlers to a variety of foods with added spices on a daily basis. We encourage you to try adding flavor to your baby's food whenever possible, whether it's homemade or store-bought. We don't mean you should add extra salt or sugar, but rather the spices you use in everyday cooking, such as garlic, curry, paprika, cinnamon, and so forth. You may find that a little spice and flavor may make food (and eating) more enjoyable for your baby.

STORE-BOUGHT BABY FOOD

If you choose to buy commercial baby food, there are many nutritious options. Here are some tips for buying the very best for your baby:

Stay away from thickening agents. Some companies dilute their foods with water and then add thickening agents, which in turn dilute the nutrients the food provides your infant. Avoid products with added sugars, starches, tapioca, rice, or other flours used to thicken.

Pay close attention to ingredients. Ingredients are listed in order by weight, so the first ingredient is the most abundant ingredient in the product. If water is the first ingredient, look to see if another brand has the actual food or foods listed first.

Look for the highest amount of nutrients. Compare different brands and choose the one with the highest amount of nutrients available per serving.

Compare calorie counts. Look at the calorie counts for single-ingredient foods. Chances are that the one with the most calories has the most food per weight

There are some organic baby foods available, such as Earth's Best, that offer a broader variety than most of the other baby-food brands, but they often cost more and may not be as readily available.

INTRODUCING MASHED FOODS

At seven or eight months of age, your baby will probably be ready to move from pureed to mashed foods. At this point your baby will likely be eating two to three meals of solid food each day. Mashed table foods are very interesting for your baby because they add more texture to meals. Some babies gag when they encounter texture changes and have trouble with this transition. If this happens to your baby, add mashed foods to her diet very slowly. To help ease the transition, you can try mixing together some baby food with real mashed foods that your family is eating. For example, mix pureed carrots or bananas with a mashed form of this food. Mix in only ½ to 1 teaspoon if your child is having trouble with the change and then gradually increase the amount of mashed food. Children who are sensitive to texture might notice small changes. You may need to start with ¼ teaspoon and give your child a few days to get used to it before increasing the amount. Soft, easy-to-mash foods include:

- sweet potatoes
- white potatoes
- carrots
- green beans
- broccoli
- cauliflower
- zucchini
- squash
- bananas
- pears
- peaches

You can use a food grinder or a food mill for tougher combination foods such as noodle dishes or ground meats. Food grinders and mills are generally available at home-goods stores and department stores like Target and Kmart.

When your baby wants to start feeding himself (usually around eight to nine months of age), give him a spoon to use while you continue to spoon food into his mouth yourself. This is called double-spooning. It allows you to continue feeding your baby while he learns a new skill. It also allows him a sense of control over eating, which can make him more inclined to eat and even try new foods. You can also start adding finger foods at this stage, such as pieces of soft fruits and vegetables, graham crackers, dry cereals, crackers, toast, pancakes or waffles, cottage cheese, or soft cheeses.

MOVING ON TO TABLE FOODS

At 10 to 12 months of age, you can expect your baby to be eating mostly table foods. After 12 months of age, he should be eating only table foods. If your baby is having trouble moving from the pureed or mashed food stage to table foods, call your pediatrician. A baby who is consuming only baby food and whole milk after his first birthday may begin to have growth problems due to inadequate calories and/or nutrients. A complete evaluation by your pediatrician and a pediatric dietitian is needed to determine the best plan to improve growth.

DID YOU KNOW?

When moving your baby to table foods, there is no need to offer him the commercially prepared toddler meals made available by many baby food manufacturers. These foods often cost two or three times what their adult counterparts cost, and they don't offer any nutritional advantage. Offering your child special meals like these can lead to short-order cooking!

TODDLERS

Toddlerhood is one of the most trying times for parents. Your child is at an age where he will do everything he can to exert his independence, which means he may begin to refuse foods that he has eaten in the past. He may also appear to "stop" eating or seem to take in significantly less food than he used to. This happens because his growth slows down dramatically after his first year, during which he likely tripled his birth weight. Toddlerhood is a time for slower growth, and your child doesn't need as much food as he used to. It's perfectly normal for toddlers to eat one meal and not eat for the rest of the day. They are often good judges of how much they should and should not eat.

However, if your toddler's growth is faltering from the growth curve or he has started refusing to eat many food groups, this is a concern. A pediatric dietitian can help you establish a schedule for meals and snacks as well as determine what nutrients your toddler may be missing as a result of the food groups he is refusing.

DID YOU KNOW?

When a child has no appetite and is failing to grow properly, he could have childhood anorexia. A relatively rare condition, childhood anorexia is characterized by extreme food refusal (eating very few or only one food or very small amounts of food), loss of appetite, and failure to thrive or grow. Improving nutrition will often improve appetite.

SCHEDULING MEALS AND SNACKS

It's important to offer toddlers food often because they have small appetites and are unable to consume large quantities at one meal. However, this does not mean that your toddler should be allowed to graze all day on foods or caloric liquids such as juice and milk. Instead, you need to set a firm schedule for when your toddler eats his meals and snacks. This will help prevent him from gaining too little weight, which can happen as a result of grazing all day long. (It's important to note that not all children who graze will have problems with weight gain, but if your child is not growing well, changing to a scheduled pattern of eating often will improve growth.) The typical food schedule for a toddler is three meals and two to three snacks a day. Spacing meals and snacks at least two hours apart—and preferably three hours apart—is recommended. Portion sizes for toddlers should be quite small—about one tablespoon of each food you are offering for every year they've been alive. So, for example, if you are having meat loaf, potatoes, and carrots for dinner, you would offer a two-year-old two tablespoons of each food. If they want seconds, that's fine.

Make sure you're offering a good variety of meals and snacks and don't let snacks turn into your toddler's favorite foods. When your toddler knows that his snack is going to be something he likes and his meal is going to be fruits and vegetables, he may fill up on snacks and refuse meals. Take Brian's story, for example. Four-year-old Brian enjoyed eating breakfast and had a good variety of foods at this meal. His lunch also often included many foods that Brian enjoyed, and he had a snack in the afternoon at preschool. Yet his mother and father reported that Brian was having a lot of trouble with dinner. He refused almost every item they fixed for him, no matter what it was, and they were cooking several meals for him every night. After we reviewed his daily food consumption, it did not appear that he was filling up on liquids or other snacks during the day. It's common for toddlers to eat only one or two good meals a day; however, Brian's behaviors at dinnertime seemed out of the ordinary. His parents had reached the point where they didn't even want to include Brian at dinner because it was "a waste of their time."

Then Brian's mom mentioned that Brian always ate a bowl of oatmeal before bedtime, sometimes two. This was his "favorite food" and he always wanted this before going to sleep. Can you see now why Brian wasn't eating dinner? He knew that in a few hours he would get his favorite food. Once we changed Brian's bedtime snack routine by varying what he was offered so that it was not so predictable, he started trying some of his dinner choices. Dinner became less of a battle. Brian's story illustrates why it's important not to make meals and snacks so routine that your toddler will know what you are going to offer. Children need one to three snacks a day, depending on their appetite. It's perfectly fine to offer food at a time when you know your toddler will reliably eat, even before bedtime, but make sure you rotate the food you offer each day. (See the sample food log on page 37 for a good example of how to schedule your child's meals, snacks, and drinks.)

SCHEDULING LIQUIDS

Many parents forget to factor liquids into their toddlers' daily feeding schedule. As you may know, drinking liquids before a meal will dampen your appetite. If your child sips on juice and milk between meals, he may not be hungry when it's time to sit down and eat. This may lead him to refuse foods and behave badly at meals. Offering liquids only with meals and snacks is a good rule of thumb. If your child is thirsty between meals, offer him sips of water instead. We recommend you limit milk to 16 to 20 ounces per day and juice to only four to six ounces per day. If your toddler has poor growth, many experts recommend that you eliminate all juice from his diet because of its high sugar content and lack of nutrition.

FOOD JAGS

Offering the same foods to your child day after day can lead to **food jags**. Food jags are periods of time (days or even weeks) when your child will eat only one or two foods. Food jags often occur during toddlerhood because the foods toddlers desire are ones they are comfortable with and know the most about. In order to prevent a food jag, you must rotate your child's favorite foods and continue to offer new foods. Allowing your child to continue on a food jag can cause him to develop a restrictive food repertoire, which puts him at risk for nutritional deficiencies and poor growth. Sara and Susan's story is a good example of this.

Two-year-old Sara and Susan were fraternal twins who had not been growing well and had a very limited food repertoire. We did a complete medical workup and found that they did not have any medical problems contributing to their feeding disorder. However, when we watched videotapes their parents made of them eating and interviewed their mother, Michelle, it became clear that the girls had a sensory processing disorder (see chapter 4 for more information) as well as behavioral issues (see chapter 5 for more information). Both girls had been hard to feed as infants and did not transition well to baby foods or table foods. Understandably, whenever the girls finally liked a food, Michelle fed it to them for every meal. When they grew tired of a food, they would switch to a different food and eat that for most meals. Their food jags began very early in life, but their parents' desire to get them to eat whatever they could made the food jags worse. In addition, both girls drank an excessive amount of liquid throughout the day. Sara drank juice and Susan drank milk. The girls were filling up on liquid and throwing major tantrums when it came time to sit down for meals.

Initially, we supported Michelle and worked on shaping the twins' behavior at mealtimes by scheduling the amount and times for liquid and food. We also rotated the girls' core diet by no longer providing their core foods every day or multiple times a day to prevent food jags and prevent more foods from falling out of their repertoire. After this was established, we implemented the food-chaining program (see chapter 6 for more information) to expand their food choices.

TIPS FOR TODDLERS' EATING SUCCESS

Here are some ways you can help ensure your toddler is getting an adequate amount of food and nutrition:

Don't stress. Growth slows down during toddlerhood, and your child's intake will vary from day to day and meal to meal. Don't stress if your child is eating only one meal a day, and don't battle him over food. It never works.

Be a good role model. If you expect your child to eat a food, offer this food often and eat it yourself.

Make them part of the fun. Bring your child food shopping with you and let him help you while you prepare meals.

No grazing. Don't allow your child to graze on food or liquid all day. Schedule meal and snack times and stick with them.

Don't short-order cook. Do not prepare your child meal after meal when he refuses to eat. End the meal and offer him a meal or snack again two to three hours later.

OLDER CHILDREN AND TEENS

Sometimes feeding problems don't become a concern until later in childhood or the teenage years. At this point parents sometimes realize that their children eat much differently than their peers, or their children may begin to stop eating foods they usually eat. Social functions can be quite stressful, and often children don't eat anything on these occasions because of their restricted food repertoire. If you haven't already done this, make your child part of food preparation and let him make some of the food decisions in the house. It can help relieve some of the stress you may be experiencing around mealtimes.

This is also the point at which you can introduce your child to basic education concepts about food. Helping your child learn about how food tastes and where it comes from, along with participating in meal decisions and preparation, will create enthusiasm to try new things.

If you have a teenager, you may be finding that his busy schedule has altered the family mealtime. Be sure to designate several meals a week where the family can be together and food can be about socialization and family culture rather than just something you child has to do before he goes to practice or to a friend's house.

Other than infancy, the teenage years mark the most rapid period of growth. Teens need more energy and therefore more nutrients. Two nutrients that are particularly important during adolescence are calcium and iron. Calcium requirements go from 800 milligrams daily to 1,300 milligrams daily to keep up with rapid growth, so make sure your teen is drinking lots of milk or getting his calcium from another source, such as cheese or yogurt. Iron is important because it helps build muscle mass. Good iron-rich foods include lean red meats, seafood, beans, and vegetables such as asparagus and broccoli. Keep in mind that girls need more iron than boys to make up for iron loss during menstruation.

FOOD ALLERGIES

As we mentioned earlier, a pediatric dietitian will examine your child for any food allergies that may be causing or contributing to her feeding problem. Food allergies are actually not as common as most people believe. They affect between 5 and 8 percent of babies under one year of age and only about 2 percent of older children. Fortunately, most children will outgrow their food allergies by the time they are three years old.

Food allergies are both hereditary and acquired. If one parent or a sibling of a child has allergies, that child has approximately a 20 to 40 percent chance of developing allergies. If both parents of a child have allergies, that child's risk increases to 40 to 60 percent. It's also possible for a child to develop food allergies even when there is no history of allergies in his family

WHAT IS A FOOD ALLERGY?

A food allergy is an adverse immunologic response to the *protein* found within a particular food, not the fat or the sugar, as many people believe. For instance, if your child has a milk allergy, he is allergic to casein and whey (the proteins found in milk), not lactose (the sugar found in milk).

Experts believe that food allergies occur when a child's immature GI tract allows large protein molecules (such as casein in milk) to enter his circulation and contact the cells of his immune system. This can cause his immune system to form antibodies for that protein. If this happens, the next time the child eats that food, he will have an allergic reaction. Children are most susceptible to this during the first three years of life, when the GI lining is highly permeable, making it easy for large protein molecules to penetrate the bloodstream. As your child grows, his GI tract matures and the junctions between the cells become tighter, preventing the passage of these larger molecules that cause allergies. This is why many health-care practitioners recommend you not introduce many common food allergens to your child's diet until he's at least one year old.

DID YOU KNOW?

Food allergies and food intolerances are not the same. A food intolerance is a chemical reaction to a particular food, not an immunological reaction, which is what an allergy is. Lactose intolerance and MSG intolerance are the most common food intolerances.

WHAT IS A FOOD INTOLERANCE?

Many people believe that a food allergy and a food intolerance are the same thing, but that is not true. Food intolerance is a digestive system response rather than an immune system response. It occurs when something in a food irritates your child's digestive system or when your child is unable to properly digest or break down a food. Here's a simple example to help explain the difference between food intolerance and allergies: if your child is lactose intolerant, he is intolerant to the lactose (also known as the sugar) found in milk. If he is allergic to milk, he is allergic to the casein or whey (also known as the protein) found in milk.

Food intolerances are much more common than food allergies. In fact, lactose intolerance, the most common food intolerance, affects about 10 percent of Americans. Intolerance symptoms tend to be milder than allergy symptoms and include nausea, stomach pain, and diarrhea, gas, cramps, bloating, vomiting, headaches, heartburn, and irritability. Unlike food allergies, which can be triggered by even a small amount of the food and occur every time the food is consumed, food intolerances may not cause symptoms unless your child eats a large portion of the food or eats the food frequently.

There are two ways to diagnose a food intolerance. The first is to keep a food log to record what your child eats and when he gets symptoms, and then look for common factors. The other way to identify problem foods is to put your child on an elimination diet. This involves completely eliminating any suspect foods from his diet until he is symptom-free. Then you reintroduce the foods to your child's diet one at a time. This can help you pinpoint which foods cause symptoms.

Treatment for food intolerance is simple—your child should either avoid problem foods altogether, or, if he displays symptoms only after consuming large quantities of a problem food, limit his consumption.

THE SEVEN COMMON FOOD ALLERGIES

Though it's possible to be allergic to just about any food, over 90 percent of food allergies, especially in young children, are caused by seven foods:

1. Milk. Cow's milk is the most common cause of food allergies. Infants who have an allergy to cow's-milk-based formulas are usually switched to a hydrolyzed formula, such as Nutramigen or Alimentum. Soy formulas and goat's milk are not good alternatives in this case, because many infants with allergies to cow's milk proteins are also allergic to the proteins in soy and goat's milk.

Other foods to avoid if your child is allergic to cow's milk include buttermilk, cheese, evaporated and condensed milk, ice cream, yogurt, instant mashed potatoes, margarine, casein, cream, hydrolysates, lactalbumin, nougat, sour cream, whey, and other foods made with milk. Older children who can't drink milk or eat milk-based foods should be sure to have additional sources of calcium in their diet and may require a calcium supplement.

2. Eggs. Eggs, especially the proteins in egg whites, are also a common cause of food allergies. If your child has an egg allergy, he needs to avoid egg substitutes and foods that contain albumin, globulin, ovalbumin, and vitellin. He should also avoid foods that are prepared with eggs, such as French toast, cake, cookies, pancakes, eggnog, bread, ice cream, pasta, puddings, creamy salad dressings, and foods with custard or cream fillings.

DID YOU KNOW?

To help prevent allergies to eggs, avoid giving eggs to infants under a year old.

3. Soybean. Soybean allergies are usually found in infants who are given a soy formula but can also be found in older children who drink soy milk. Other foods that contain soy proteins and may cause allergic symptoms in children allergic to soy include tofu, miso soup, soy sauce, foods prepared in soybean oil, veggie burgers and hot dogs, and ingredients such as emulsifiers and hydrolyzed or textured vegetable protein.

DID YOU KNOW?

Even if your child has a soy allergy, he may not need to avoid soybean oil, because the oil does not contain the protein that causes a soy allergy. However, some cold-pressed or extruded soybean oils do get cross-contaminated, so be sure to ask your child's pediatrician if soybean oil is OK for him to consume (see page 74 for more information on avoiding **cross-contamination**).

4. Wheat. Wheat allergy can develop in infants given a wheat cereal, so we recommend offering a rice or oat cereal first and to delay giving wheat until after your child is six to eight months old. If your child has a wheat allergy, he should avoid all breads and cereals made with wheat flour or enriched flour. He can, however, eat bread and cereals made from oats, rye, corn, or rice. Your child should also avoid foods containing cornstarch, gluten, semolina, all-purpose flour, and white flour.

5. Peanuts. Peanuts are not true nuts—they are actually legumes from the pea and bean family. Children with a peanut allergy can be very sensitive to foods with even very small amounts of peanuts in them. If your child has a peanut allergy, he should avoid all foods with peanuts, including candy, baked goods, chili, many ethnic foods (including Thai, Asian, and Indonesian foods), peanut butter, and mixed nuts.

> **DID YOU KNOW?**
>
> Children who are allergic to peanuts can often eat tree nuts such as walnuts or pecans, since they are from separate plant families. Just make sure the nuts are not processed in the same place as peanuts to avoid cross-contamination.

6. Tree Nuts. Tree nuts include walnuts, pecans, cashews, almonds, hazelnuts, and other nuts in hard shells. If your child is allergic to tree nuts, he should avoid foods prepared with them, including many kinds of candy, baked goods, and different oils.

7. Shellfish. The shellfish commonly known to cause allergic reactions include shrimp, crab, crayfish, lobster, oysters, clams, scallops, mussels, squid, and snails. Read food labels carefully if your child is allergic to shellfish, because highly processed foods may contain hidden fish or shellfish. For example, the basis for imitation crab, lobster, and shrimp is pollack. It can also be used in beef and pork substitutes and as part of hot dogs, ham, and pizza toppings.

FOOD ALLERGY SYMPTOMS

Symptoms of a food allergy include wheezing and difficulty breathing, itchy skin rashes (such as hives and eczema), vomiting, diarrhea, nausea, abdominal pain, and swelling around your child's mouth and in his throat. These symptoms usually develop fairly quickly after your child eats the food he is allergic to, usually within minutes to hours. Nasal symptoms by themselves, such as congestion or a runny nose, are usually not caused by food allergies.

Food allergy symptoms may be mild or very severe, depending on how much of the food your child ingested and how allergic he is to the food. A severe reaction can include anaphylaxis, which is characterized by difficulty breathing, swelling in the mouth and throat, decreased blood pressure, shock, and even death.

DIAGNOSING FOOD ALLERGIES

The best way to determine whether your child is allergic to a food is to eliminate that food from his diet for two weeks and watch him to see if his symptoms resolve themselves (also known as an elimination diet). To test your findings, you can reintroduce a suspected allergen into your child's diet to see if he exhibits any allergy symptoms. If you have an infant, you can switch him to a soy, protein hydrolysate, or elemental (amino acid) formula for a week or two to see if his symptoms disappear.

Your pediatrician or pediatric dietitian may also recommend that your child see an allergist for further evaluation. There is no single test available to diagnose a food allergy, but the following tests may help pinpoint what food allergy your child has:

Skin test. A skin test is helpful in uncovering hidden food allergies, but it has a high incidence of false positives, meaning the skin test is likely to show that your child is allergic to a food when really he is not. However, a negative skin test (i.e., your child does not react to a certain food allergen injected in his skin) is a reliable indication that he is not allergic to that food.

Blood test. This test, called a RAST (Radio-allergo-sorbent test), measures the antibodies in your child's bloodstream to certain food allergens. Unlike the skin test, a RAST test has a high degree of false negatives, meaning it often does not detect food allergies that your child really has. A positive RAST test is a reliable indicator that your child is allergic to that food. If a certain food, say, peanuts, shows up positive on a RAST test, that means your child is more likely than not to be allergic to peanuts. If a skin test and a RAST test agree, the results carry even more weight.

FOOD ALLERGIES CAN SOMETIMES BE PREVENTED

Studies show that there are steps you can take to prevent your child from developing food allergies:

- Avoid peanut butter during pregnancy.
- Breast-feed exclusively for the first six months of your baby's life (that means no formula supplements or solid foods) and then continue to breast-feed until your child is at least 12 months old.
- Avoid peanuts and tree nuts while breast-feeding. Also consider avoiding eggs, cow's milk, and fish while nursing.
- If you do want to supplement your breast-feeding

with formula, use a hypoallergenic formula, such as Nutramigen or Alimentum.

- Do not introduce solid foods to your infant until he is at least six months old, and then start with an iron-fortified rice cereal.
- Avoid feeding your child milk and dairy products until he is 12 months old.
- Avoid introducing eggs (especially egg whites) until he is two years old.
- Avoid peanuts, tree nuts, and fish until he is three years old.

LIVING WITH A FOOD ALLERGY

If it has been confirmed that your child has a food allergy, you must eliminate all foods containing the allergen from his diet. Reading food labels is the key to avoiding allergens, because food protein can be hidden in many different sources. For example, some nondairy foods contain milk, and peanuts can be found in some barbecue sauces.

READ FOOD LABELS

Potentially allergenic foods may be listed under another name in packaged foods. The most common are:

- wheat flour: durum semolina, farina
- egg white: albumin
- dairy products: casein, sodium caseinate

Carefully reading labels will help you discover what your child is eating:

- Cocoa mixes, creamed foods, gravies, and some sauces contain milk.
- Noodles and pasta contain wheat and sometimes eggs.
- Canned soups may contain wheat and dairy fillers.
- Most breads contain wheat and dairy products.
- Margarine usually contains whey.
- Hot dogs, cold cuts, and "nondairy" desserts contain sodium caseinate.

Avoiding cross-contamination in your home is also an important part of preventing allergic reactions. Cross-contamination is the contamination of a food product from another source. For instance, if you use a knife to butter a piece of bread that contains wheat and then the same knife is reinserted into the butter, the butter may now contain traces of wheat and is therefore contaminated. Someone with a wheat allergy could have an allergic reaction if he uses that butter or the same knife to butter another food. You should always cook allergen-free foods first, before using the pan to cook a food that contains allergens that could affect your child. It's also a good idea to designate a special shelf or cupboard for "safe" foods, and you might consider buying your child his own toaster if he has a wheat allergy.

STAYING HEALTHY

It's important for your child to see a pediatric dietitian to make sure his "allergy-proof" diet is nutritionally sound. If your child has to avoid foods or food groups, there is a greater potential for him to be deficient in certain vitamins and minerals. There are many food substitutes the dietitian can suggest to replace the food that your child needs to avoid. For example, eggs can be replaced by a mixture of baking powder, water, and vinegar in a recipe. Rice milk could be used in place of cow's milk. (The Resources section on page 357 has helpful information for families living with food allergies.)

Making sure that your child receives the right nutrition is critical to his health and well-being, and now you're armed with the information and guidelines you need to ensure that this happens. Food allergies can also play a role in eating problems, so watch your child for any of the signs we've discussed in this chapter that may indicate he's got an allergy. In the next chapter, we discuss your child's eating and swallowing skills and the role they play in eating problems.

CHAPTER 3

Does My Child Have a Problem with Eating Skills?

The Feeding Evaluation

Amy and Brian were concerned that their two-month-old daughter Mia didn't seem to know how to take her bottle. They worried she wasn't getting enough food—formula spilled from her mouth and her burp cloth was very wet by the end of each feeding. Mia seemed congested when she took her bottle and she coughed at times. It took Mia a long time to drink just a few ounces. She would fall asleep or just seem too tired to continue.

Mia started to have frequent colds and occasional fevers and she was hospitalized a few times for upper respiratory problems. Her doctor was concerned that she had reflux and put her on medicine, but it didn't seem to help. Mia's weight gain was poor.

Amy and Brian took Mia to a long list of specialists who evaluated their daughter, and finally, a ***pulmonologist*** *recommended that they take Mia to a speech therapist for a swallowing evaluation. There, the speech therapist also administered a test called a* ***modified barium swallow study,*** *which was like a moving X-ray of Mia while she ate. It turned out that small amounts of the formula were going "the wrong way" down Mia's airway instead of down to her stomach. When the therapist changed the nipple to a slower-flowing product and changed Mia's position while she ate, she had a much easier time taking her bottle.*

However, the therapist was still worried about Mia's poor growth, very low energy level, and fatigue while eating. The therapist contacted Mia's pediatrician and requested a consult with a dietitian, who put Mia on a higher-calorie formula. Amy and Brian took Mia to weekly therapy sessions with the speech therapist to improve her feeding skills, and she had periodic checkups with the dietitian. Today, at age 11 months, she is thriving and eating normally.

MANY PEOPLE DON'T know this, but we use the same muscles and structures of the face to speak and to eat. Your child may have a physical problem, or an oral motor skill issue, such as difficulty sucking, swallowing, biting, chewing, or coordinating tongue movements, that interferes with her ability to eat an appropriate diet safely. A speech therapist is trained to help children with speech problems and feeding disorders that pertain to oral motor skills and swallowing. He will observe a meal and complete a full food analysis, which involves looking at what your child eats well and why. He'll determine which utensils your child should be using and the right bottles and nipples or cups for her liquid intake. He will also select the safest consistency of liquid for your child to consume. The speech therapist is also typically the one who is primarily responsible for developing and updating your child's food chains. However, in some regions, this may be done by the dietitian or the occupational therapist.

In this chapter, we discuss what to expect at the speech therapist appointment, the tests and procedures he may use to assess your child's eating problems, and how he will help your child overcome them. You will learn about the role oral motor skills play in your child's ability to eat properly and the symptoms your child might exhibit if she has a problem. You'll also learn about the mechanics of a swallow and how to recognize whether your child is having trouble swallowing. Finally, we guide you through the process of choosing the eating equipment (nipples, bottles, spoons, cups, and so forth) best suited to your child's needs.

SIGNS THAT YOUR CHILD MAY HAVE AN ORAL MOTOR SKILL OR SWALLOWING PROBLEM

If your baby or older child exhibits one or more of the following signs, she may be having trouble with the oral motor skills involved in eating, or she may have a swallowing problem:

- loud, gulpy swallows
- gurgling sound when swallowing
- coughing

- wide eyes or raised eyebrows
- a "distressed" appearance
- watery eyes while drinking or eating
- congestion that increases as feeding progresses
- weak suck (your baby seems fatigued when sucking)
- poor suck (your baby isn't using the muscles of the lips, tongue, and cheek well)
- inability to hold pacifier in mouth
- formula spilling from the mouth
- fatigue as feeding progresses
- color change when eating (white or blue around the mouth and eyes)
- breathing only through the mouth
- refusal of food
- need to swallow multiple times in order to swallow one bite of food
- poor chewing ability (i.e., your child spits food out, doesn't chew well enough, or swallows food whole without chewing it)
- food is left in the mouth after swallowing or remains "pocketed" in between the teeth and inner cheek
- heavy drooling, to the point where you need to change her shirt frequently or use a bib
- taking of only a few ounces of liquid and then ceasing to drink
- labored breathing when eating
- "panting" respiration patterns when eating
- gagging while eating

- frequent illness, such as colds, congestion, upper respiratory infection, fevers of unexplained origin, and asthma that does not improve with treatment
- snoring, poor sleep patterns, and breathing through the mouth while sleeping

DID YOU KNOW?

One of the common myths about eating is that it is easy and instinctive. Eating is actually the most complex physical task humans engage in. It is the only physical task that utilizes all of the body's organ systems: the brain and cranial nerves; the heart and vascular system; the respiratory, endocrine, and metabolic systems; all the muscles of the body; and the entire GI tract. Swallowing alone requires the coordination of 26 muscles and six cranial nerves.

—Kay Toomey, PhD, Director of Colorado Pediatric Therapy and Feeding Specialists

THE SPEECH THERAPY APPOINTMENT

After the pediatric dietitian has completed his examination of your child and created a nutritional care plan to meet her needs, it's time to visit a speech therapist for a feeding evaluation. If you need to find a speech therapist for your child, first ask her current health-care practitioners for referrals. The dietitian in particular may work closely with one or more speech therapists and could make some reliable recommendations. You can also find a therapist through ProSearch on the American Speech-Language-Hearing Association (ASHA) Web site at www.asha.org. Be sure to select a speech therapist who is certified, credentialed, and very experienced in oral motor/ feeding therapy with children. You can tell if a speech therapist is properly qualified if he has CCC/SLP after his name. This means he has a certificate of clinical competency and has passed the certification examination. You should feel comfortable with the therapist and his philosophy and approach to feeding, and your child should also feel comfortable in treatment. If this is not the case, don't hesitate to try another therapist. Your child will do best working with someone she likes and someone you trust.

The first thing the speech therapist will do during your visit is take a thorough medical history of your child. There are certain symptoms that the therapist is looking for in your child's history that will help him pinpoint whether her oral motor skills are causing or contributing to her feeding problem. Oral motor skills are the mechanical skills your child needs to master in order to eat properly. For instance, babies must be able to make forward and backward tongue movements in order to breast- or bottle-feed. They must learn to close their lips around the spoon to help draw the food into the mouth and cup their tongue to move food to the back of their mouth in order to spoon-feed successfully. In order to manage the transition to table foods, babies need to learn how to move the tongue to the sides of the mouth and place a bite of food onto the molar area of the gums. To drink from a cup, they need to learn how to hold a small amount of fluid in the mouth and to pull it into a ball (or bolus) for swallowing. If your child has a problem with these or any other oral motor skills, it is certainly playing a role in how she eats. The therapist will pay particularly close attention to signs that your child may have dysphagia, or a problem with swallowing.

You can also expect the therapist to evaluate your child's oral reflexes (root, suck, swallow, gag, bite, and her ability to move her tongue toward the side of her mouth). He will determine if your child's oral motor skills match up with the method by which she is being fed and make any necessary changes. This usually involves recommendations for a different bottle, nipple, cup, or spoon better suited to your child's needs.

After he has evaluated your child, the speech therapist will discuss his findings with your pediatrician and start her on a feeding program. However, if your child has dysphagia, she will likely require additional evaluation before she can begin a program.

WHAT IS DYSPHAGIA?

Dysphagia means "difficulty swallowing." It is when food or liquids do not pass easily from the mouth, into the throat, and down into the esophagus to the stomach during the process of swallowing. To understand dysphagia, you must first understand the mechanics of a swallow.

Swallowing is a complex, three-stage process. These three stages are controlled by nerves that connect the digestive tract to the brain. The first stage is called the oral preparation stage. This is when food is chewed and moistened by saliva. The tongue pushes food and liquids to the back of the mouth toward the throat. (This phase is voluntary: we have control over chewing and beginning to swallow.)

Next is the pharyngeal stage. Food enters the pharynx, which is the area inside the mouth where food leaves the tongue and enters the throat. The pharynx extends from up behind the nose to behind the mouth and has sensory receptors that tell the brain there is something there to swallow. The swallow should trigger in about one second. The timing of the swallow reflex is the key to a safe swallow. A flap called the **epiglottis** closes off the passage to the windpipe so food cannot get into the lungs. The muscles in the throat relax. Food and liquid are quickly passed down the pharynx into the esophagus. The epiglottis opens again so we can breathe. (This phase starts under voluntary control, but then becomes an involuntary phase that we cannot consciously control.)

Last is the esophageal stage. Liquids fall through the esophagus into the stomach by gravity. Muscles in the esophagus push food toward the stomach in wavelike movements known as peristalsis. A muscular band between the end of the esophagus and the upper portion of the esophagus relaxes in response to swallowing, allowing food and liquids to enter the stomach. (The events in this phase are involuntary.)

A swallowing disorder occurs when one or more of these stages do not take place properly.

ISAAC'S STORY

Four-month-old Isaac's parents brought him to see us because he was frequently choking during bottle feedings. He had been diagnosed with pneumonia at two months of age and again at four months, and he was on twice-a-day breathing treatments for wheezing, but otherwise he was in normal health. During the initial evaluation, we saw that an excessive amount of formula was spilling out of the corners of his mouth while he drank, causing him to cough immediately. A test confirmed he was indeed aspirating small amounts of formula into his lungs. It turned out that Isaac was drinking from a fast-flow nipple that his family bought because it was taking so long for him to finish a bottle. During his feeding evaluation, we also discovered that Isaac was not sealing his lips around the nipple well, and his sucking was weak.

After switching Isaac to a medium-flow Gerber nipple and thickening his formula slightly, he no longer aspirated formula into his lungs and was able to swallow safely. No formula came out of the sides of his mouth while he was drinking. We also showed Isaac's parents how to position him upright while he was taking his bottle and recommended therapy to improve Isaac's lip seal around the nipple and improve the strength of his suck. It was very important to make sure Isaac felt safe during feedings (choking on formula makes babies feel very unsafe) because if he didn't, he might begin to refuse feedings, which would negatively affect his growth and development. It's also important to solve infant feeding problems such as Isaac's as early as possible, because babies must master bottle-feeding (or breast-feeding) skills in order to reach the next step in feeding, which is clearing food off a spoon.

THE FEEDING HISTORY

Next, the speech therapist will do an evaluation of your child's feeding history. He may interview you on the phone during the scheduling process, or you may receive a form with questions about your child's ability to eat. The therapist will likely go over many of these questions again during the evaluation. This history is very important—each stage of feeding affects the next, and the therapist needs to have an idea of what has contributed to your child's feeding problem in order to provide effective treatment. In order to get as complete a history as possible, the therapist will likely ask you some or all of the following questions:

- Where does your child prefer to eat? In your lap, a high chair, a booster seat, or a chair at the kitchen table? Or does she prefer to eat while standing or walking around?
- If your child eats her meals in a high chair, does the tray seem too high or too tight?
- Where is your child positioned after feeding? For instance, if you have an infant, do you typically put her in her car seat or an infant swing after she's done eating? Do you hold her in your lap? Put her on the floor? Is she in an upright or reclined position?

- Can your child sit up and support her upper body well, or does she slouch when in a seated position?
- Is there adequate support under your child's feet when she's eating? (Her feet need support in order to make the best possible use of her body as well as the muscles involved in chewing and swallowing while eating.)
- Can your child maintain a good, stable neck position? (Her neck should not be hyperextended.)

The therapist will use this information to determine the best way to position your child so that her body is properly supported and the muscles of her head, neck, and face work best. The repositioning of a child to eat is a major part of the treatment program. A change in position helps the child have better control of food and liquid in the mouth. Many issues can be resolved solely with positioning changes.

The therapist will also ask you questions about the environment in which your child eats her meals:

- What is the environment for a typical meal in your home? Noisy or quiet? Stressful or calm?
- Does your child have a hard time eating in a noisy or busy environment? Does she need quiet when she eats?
- How does your child approach a mealtime setting? Is she eager, or does she require coaxing? Does she refuse to sit down to eat? Does she cry?

- Does your child tolerate eating better when she feeds herself?
- How does your child approach food? (For instance, does she approach food with fear or anxiety? Does she move away from the table or avoid mealtimes? Does she appear hungry and motivated to eat or show no sign of appetite?)
- Does she tolerate food on her hands and face?
- In your opinion, how efficient are her fine motor skills? Can she use utensils well? Grasp her drinking cup?
- How does your child tolerate being fed by you or another caregiver?

The therapist will use this information to make recommendations for changes to your child's feeding environment. Your child may eat better in low light or with less noise from the television or from conversation. Soft instrumental music at meals may also be helpful.

If your child pulls her hands away from a plate, touches food with one finger, or wipes her hands on her shirt frequently while eating, she may eat better using utensils and with a wet washcloth beside the plate. The therapist will help you choose foods your child can touch without distress. He will also provide activities to help reduce the sensitivity of your child's hands and improve her touch tolerance for a variety of textures.

Sensory preparation before meals is also very important.

Some children do well with a sensory activity prior to eating such as blowing on kazoos, whistle straws, or other music toys, singing and marching to the dinner table, and jumping or bouncing on a therapy ball. Then the child is transitioned to the table and the therapist will make sure she is well supported while feeding. He will help you find ways in all eating environments to provide good support under your child's feet and to the pelvis so she feels secure and can use the muscles of the face and mouth well while eating.

You will also be asked questions about your child's meal schedule, or the timing of her meals:

- How many minutes does it take for your child to complete a meal?
- Does your child appear to be hungry at meal and snack times?
- Does your child graze on food (nibble or snack throughout the day)?
- Does your child have a schedule by which she eats her meals and snacks and drinks her liquids?

The therapist will use this information as well as the information he will glean from the questions below to determine if your child's meals and snacks can be scheduled to gently enhance her appetite and to see if his oral motor skills are adequate to meet her needs orally. If meals last too long, your child may not have the ability or the energy to take in enough food by mouth.

The therapist will need to know specifics about your child's oral motor skills. She will evaluate these areas herself, but she will also ask you questions about your child's skills. The therapist will likely ask the following:

- Is your child able to completely close her lips on a nipple or spoon, and can she maintain a lip seal while bottle-/breast-feeding or chewing?
- How would you describe your child's feeding skills? Is your child able to chew a bite of food and gather it together in the middle of her mouth for swallowing? (If there are problems, you may observe food pocketing in her mouth or inside her cheeks.)
- Does your child seem to lose control of food or liquid in her mouth before or during the swallow?
- Can you describe the type of chewing pattern she has? There are two main patterns: the munching pattern and the rotary chewing pattern. The munching pattern is an up-and-down type of munch, where your child doesn't really rotate her jaw. This is a more primitive pattern of chewing. The rotary chewing pattern is the more mature pattern. Rotary chewing allows your child to move food under her teeth and move her tongue more efficiently to transfer a bite of food from the molars to the tongue before swallowing.
- Can your child move her tongue to the sides of her mouth to move food around in her mouth?

- Can she lift her tongue to her palate?
- Can your child cup her tongue to control liquid or food in her mouth?

The therapist will use this information to pick the right feeding products based on your child's motor skills. He will also determine what type of therapy program your child needs to strengthen and improve the function of the muscles of his face and mouth. Your answers to these questions can also indicate whether your child may have a swallow problem.

The therapist will want to know about your child's respiration, or breathing, before, during, and after her meals:

- Do you hear your child making gulpy swallows? Is she congested while eating?
- Do you observe her gagging, coughing, or choking while she's swallowing?
- Do you have any concerns about your child's swallowing skills?
- Before your child eats, is her breathing clear?
- Does her breathing become gurgly when she eats?
- Does your child demonstrate "wet" breathing patterns? (A "wet" breathing pattern would be if your child appears to be breathing normally, but when she starts eating you can literally hear the congestion and collection of liquid or food in her throat. Infants may also have a rattle in their chest.)

- Does your child cough during meals?
- After she eats, is your child's breathing clear, gurgly, or wet? Is she panting?

Like the information above, your answers here will help the therapist assess whether your child is swallowing properly and safely.

DID YOU KNOW?

It's normal for babies to gag themselves with mouthing toys. They are actually desensitizing their gag reflex, which allows them to move to the next stage of feeding. A gag is triggered on the front of an infant's tongue to protect her from putting an item into her mouth that she could choke on. As a baby mouths toys and gags herself, she is moving the gag trigger farther back on her tongue. This is why an adult's gag reflex triggers far back in the throat.

The therapist will also likely ask your opinion on:

- How efficiently your child swallows her food and drink.
- Whether your child needs to swallow multiple times to clear her throat. If so, how many swallows are necessary?
- Whether you can audibly hear your child breathing after she swallows.

Finally, the therapist will ask you whether your child has mastered the following feeding methods and if you have any concerns about them:

- Drinking from a bottle
- Drinking from a cup (What type of cup? A sippy cup or an open cup?)
- Drinking from a straw
- Spoon feeding (What type of spoon does she use?)
- Finger feeding
- Using utensils

Every feeding skill builds upon the ones that come before it, so it's important for the therapist to pinpoint where the process may have broken down for your child. Your answers to these questions will help him do just that, as well as give him the information he needs to make specific recommendations regarding your child's bottle, cup, and spoon, if necessary.

THE PHYSICAL EXAM

The physical examination is a very important part of the speech therapist's evaluation. Some children are resistant to this part of the process, but an experienced therapist will be able to put your child at ease and recognize and respect the sensory issues that may be creating her anxiety. He'll start by looking in your child's mouth to check the structures and the alignment of her teeth, and to see if enlarged tonsils are possibly affecting the swallow. The therapist will also evaluate your child's ability to move her tongue and the muscles of her cheeks and lips with and without food in her mouth. He may implement a play-based evaluation using dolls or puppets that eat during this portion of the exam and have your child act out dinnertime at home or show her how she will listen to your child swallow (see cervical auscultation on page 95 for more information). The therapist should explain each step of the process in language your child understands.

THE FEEDING OBSERVATION

The therapist will also want to observe your child both eating food and drinking liquid and evaluate her responses. If you are bottle-feeding your infant, the therapist will evaluate how your baby is positioned for bottle-feeding, the nipple you use, and how fast liquid flows into her mouth. Based on his findings, the therapist may change the nipple you're using for a new one that allows your baby to have better control of the liquid in her mouth during swallowing. The therapist may also change your baby's positioning to help her have more control while swallowing. He will also evaluate how much energy your child uses to eat and determine how efficient your child is at coordinating the suck/swallow/breathe sequence (see chapter 4 for an in-depth discussion on this).

If your child has already moved on to solid foods, the therapist will observe how you offer your baby food, how you and your child communicate during a meal, and whether you and your child are generally "in sync" during meals. The therapist may suggest that you slow down the pace of the meal, adding

> **HELPFUL HINT**
>
> It's a good idea to provide a videotape of your child eating a meal in her home environment that the speech therapist can view prior to your child's appointment. The videotape will provide your child's therapist with significant insight into her feeding environment and allow him to view your child when she's most comfortable and uninhibited.

more time between bites of baby food to allow your child to swallow in between bites or give her smaller bites of food. He will also evaluate the position in which your child typically eats to see if it needs adjustment.

If your child has reached the stage where she is feeding herself, the therapist will observe how well your child uses her hands and utensils to bring food to her mouth. The therapist will also observe how well your child tolerates food on her hands or face. Based on his findings, the therapist may suggest that you change the size or type of utensils your child is using. Your child's cup and straw drinking skills will also be evaluated, and you may be instructed to thicken the liquids your child drinks to help her swallow them safely.

During the feeding observation, the therapist may use a technique called **cervical auscultation** to listen to your child swallow while she is eating and drinking. During cervical auscultation, the therapist will place a stethoscope on the side of your child's neck to listen to the timing and effectiveness of her swallow reflex. There are two sounds the therapist is listening for: the opening of the **eustachian tube** and opening of the upper esophageal sphincter. A bite of food or sip of liquid should clear your child's throat easily in one swallow, and a cervical auscultation will help the therapist determine if this is happening as it should. If the therapist has any lingering concerns regarding the safety of your child's swallow, he will recommend either a modified barium swallow study (also known as a cookie swallow) or a **fiberoptic endoscopic evaluation of the swallow (FEES).** These tests are completed to rule out the possibility your child might aspirate food or liquid into her airway. Your therapist will recommend the procedure that will best provide information for your child.

MODIFIED BARIUM SWALLOW STUDY

A modified barium swallow study (also known as a cookie swallow and a video oral pharyngeal swallow study [VOSS] or video fluoroscopic swallow study [VFSS]) is very similar to an upper GI series (see chapter 1 for more information). Cervical auscultation and observation reveal a limited amount of information, and a swallow study will ensure that your child's swallow is safe.

The speech therapist, along with a radiologist, will be present and may videotape the study for further review after the study is over. Basically, the study involves watching your child eat a meal, and the speech therapist and radiologist will want to mimic a typical feeding situation for your child as closely as possible so they can study her typical swallowing pattern. To this end, you may be asked to bring your child's own bottle, spoon, cup, and so forth and possibly some of the foods and drinks your child typically has at home. Barium will be mixed into various foods and drinks so it will not taste unpleasant. (Barium can be mixed into juices, baby food, chocolate milk, puddings, dips, spaghetti sauces, or cream soups, or even put on a sandwich, to name a few possibilities). If the food tastes acceptable to your child, you are much more likely to get a good study. In most cases, you will be asked to feed your child or stand in front of her while she self-feeds. We do not advocate using a syringe or a forced approach to complete a study. In many facilities, a child life specialist will be present to work with the therapist and radiologist to help your child feel comfortable during the study.

The speech therapist and radiologist will then watch your child swallow various textures of foods and thin liquids (and possibly thicker liquids if necessary). They are looking for signs of a problem in the way she prepares the foods and liquids in her mouth to swallow them, and with the swallow itself. They are also looking for signs that your child is aspirating foods or liquids into her lungs when she eats. When the study is completed, the team will likely review it again on videotape in slow motion. Trace aspiration can be missed unless there are two reviewers evaluating the study frame by frame. The team should also allow you to observe the study, explain the findings to you, and answer any of your questions.

FIBEROPTIC ENDOSCOPIC EVALUATION OF THE SWALLOW (FEES)

Some therapists recommend a FEES study instead of a modified barium swallow study. In a FEES study, a small flexible fiberoptic endoscope (a small tube with a miniature camera and light on the end of it) is used to view your child's pharynx (throat) and larynx (voice box). The inside of your child's nose is coated with an anesthetic gel to reduce the sensation of the endoscope being passed. The endoscope is passed through her nose to a position slightly above the voice box. Once your child is comfortable, she will be given foods or liquids that are tinted with food dye so the speech therapist can follow their passage.

As with the modified barium swallow study, the therapist will watch your child prepare the foods and liquids in her mouth to swallow them and she will carefully observe your child's swallow to make sure food and liquid pass safely to the esophagus. Important aspects such as the speed of the swallow, the amount of food or liquid that is not swallowed on the first swallow, and the amounts of foods or liquids that drop near or into the airway are also observed. At the same time, the entire examination is videotaped so that the therapist, as well as other members of your child's feeding team, can view the results as often as necessary and offer a treatment plan.

These tests may sound intimidating, but if your child does require one, take comfort in the fact that you will find out exactly what foods and liquids she can safely eat and how to work to improve her feeding and swallowing skills.

CHOOSING YOUR CHILD'S EATING EQUIPMENT

When you go into a baby goods store like Babies "R" Us and you look at the wall where the bottles, nipples, cups, spoons, and bowls are displayed, it's difficult to know what to buy. There are literally hundreds of different styles and types of feeding products to choose from, each with its own purpose and special properties. Most parents don't know enough about what each product is designed to do to make an informed decision about which ones to buy. Here is some advice on choosing the best supplies to suit your child's needs.

CHOOSING A PACIFIER

When choosing a pacifier for your baby, look for one that is similar in shape to a bottle nipple. A long and narrow-shaped pacifier will encourage correct tongue placement, tongue grooving, and cheek-muscle activation when your baby is sucking. A pacifier that is too short will not provide your baby with enough input to her tongue. Her tongue may actually get caught behind the nipple, which will result in poor sucking. A pacifier that is wide and flat will encourage your baby's tongue to flatten rather than groove and cup. Your baby must learn to groove and cup the tongue in order to begin bottle-feeding, otherwise she won't be able to control liquid in her mouth. Soothie brand pacifiers are our favorite and are available at most baby stores.

CHOOSING A NIPPLE

The right nipple is critical to your baby's success at sucking and swallowing. All nipples are not created equal. Some nipples flow when the baby pauses to breathe and swallow. Some nipples are difficult to suck liquid out of. Others are too short, and the baby's tongue is not placed correctly for good sucking. Still others flow too fast, overwhelming the baby with formula or breast milk when she attempts to suck.

We recommend a standard-shaped nipple, such as a Gerber or Evenflo nipple, that helps babies learn to cup the tongue around the nipple. This will help your baby keep the liquid from spreading out all through the inside of her mouth. Tongue cupping is how we collect a bite of food or liquid together and move it to the back of the throat to be swallowed in one cohesive unit. This is a vital skill for learning to eat well.

The flow rate of the nipple is critical to feeding success. Most nipples come in several different flow rates, from preemie to stage III flow. Unless you have a preemie, it is often recommended you begin with a stage I nipple. Do note that most premature babies who are having problems feeding need a speech therapist assessment to determine what feeding product is best for them. If you try a nipple and you see liquid spilling from your baby's mouth, it may mean that your baby is not able to keep up with the rate of flow from the nipple, so you should try a slower flow rate (i.e., switch from a stage II flow rate nipple to a stage I nipple and see if that works). If you're looking for a specific brand recommendation, ask your baby's speech pathologist or occupational therapist what products she suggests for your baby. Be prepared for some trial and error. You may have to go through one, two, even three different types of nipple before you find the right one for your baby. Be sure to give your baby some time to adjust to a new nipple. It may take 24 to 36 hours before she feels comfortable with a nipple change. If your baby is coughing, choking, or having other obvious problems, contact your therapist or physician.

CHOOSING A SPOON

When looking for a spoon, you will find both soft- and hard-bowl spoons. Soft-bowl spoons are better accepted by children who do not like to have something hard in their mouths. Other children like hard-bowl spoons because they prefer a firm surface against their tongue. A hard-bowl spoon helps them position their tongues correctly and enables them to better clear the food from the spoon. When you are shopping, you will find spoons that have a square-shaped bowl while others are rounded; some are narrow and some are wide. Keep in mind the size of your child's mouth when choosing a spoon and match the product to your child so it can be placed comfortably on the front part of her tongue, where she accepts food. Also consider the depth of the bowl of the spoon. You're looking for a spoon that your child can clean food off by bringing her top lip down and taking the food off the spoon. You don't want to have to scrape the food into her mouth. If the bowl of the spoon is too deep, you may be inclined to angle the spoon and scrape it against the roof of your child's mouth to clear the spoon completely.

CHOOSING A CUP

You should take the same care in choosing the right sippy cup as you did in choosing the right nipple. There are many different types of sippy cups—some have a hard spout, others have a soft one. Some have valves, others don't. Some spouts are broad and thin, others are soft and square-shaped. You want the cup to have a spout that your baby can easily seal her lips around and that does not flow too rapidly. You can determine how fast a particular cup flows by drinking from the cup yourself. Your baby's therapists can help you judge which cup is right for her. Nuby and Dr. Brown's cups are our favorites.

The bottom line is that no child should start a feeding program without a feeding evaluation by a speech therapist. This step protects your child and reduces her risk for aspiration or choking. After completing this step of treatment you can rest easy knowing that your child can safely start food chaining. In the next chapter, we discuss the sensory side of eating. There you will learn how your child tolerates the visual appearance, aromas, and feeling of food on her hands and inside her mouth. The sensory evaluation will reveal information about how to help your child tolerate new foods and sensations so she can start expanding her diet and learn how to enjoy eating again (or, for some children, for the first time).

CHAPTER 4

Why Does My Child Refuse Certain Foods?

The Sensory Evaluation

Molly, mother of four-year-old Jim, has always been worried about her son's development and feeding skills. As a baby, his muscles were weak and he was late to roll, sit, crawl, and walk. When he drank from his bottle, he gagged easily, spit up frequently, and would allow only his parents or his grandparents (who visited frequently) to feed him. When Molly started Jim on baby foods, he was picky and would gag easily, occasionally to the point of vomiting. When she transitioned him to table foods, Jim began vomiting in response to certain textures and smells.

When Jim became a toddler, Molly noticed that he avoided activities that other boys seemed to enjoy, especially the messy ones, like stomping in mud puddles, using finger paints, and playing with slime. As he grew older, it became clear to Molly that Jim was uncoordinated, had difficulty making transitions from one activity to another, had a hard time following directions, and had trouble making friends. He just didn't seem to be adapting normally and looked "lost" in the world of play. On top of this, Jim would eat very few foods—only french fries, plain McDonald's hamburgers, Wendy's chicken nuggets, Cheetos, the cheese and crust from pizza, ice cream, chocolate milk, juice, and soda.

Jim starts school next year, and Molly is becoming increasingly anxious about how he will handle the pressures, from eating in the cafeteria to dealing with a messy classroom activity. She's just not sure how to help him.

THINK OF A food item that you dislike or refuse to eat. Imagine you've been told that you have to eat every last piece of it and you have to use your hands to feed yourself—no utensils. Can you imagine eating that food when you cannot even handle touching it? How much stress does the thought of doing this cause you? Are you sweating or feeling nauseous? Have you suddenly lost your appetite?

This is what children with a sensory processing disorder go through every time they are confronted with a food they don't consider "safe." Children with a sensory processing disorder often have a difficult time touching, let alone manipulating, food. This is why these kids tend to accept only a few foods—these are the foods they can handle from a sensory perspective.

WHAT IS SENSORY PROCESSING?

Every second of every day we are bombarded with sensory input from the world around us. It's impossible for us to process everything we see, hear, touch, taste, and smell in a given day, so our brains filter the essential information from the irrelevant. This is called sensory processing, or the way in which the brain interprets, organizes, and uses sensory information. When the brain is able to process relevant sensory information, we respond efficiently and automatically. But when there is a disruption in the intake and organization of sensory input, this affects our ability to recognize and respond to sensory information in an appropriate manner.

Exposure to sensory stimuli begins while we are in the womb and continues throughout our adult life. As we mature with an efficient neurological system, we are able to filter the multiple sensory messages around us. When problems occur, such as a sensory processing disorder, it affects children in every area of their lives, including feeding. Different affected sensory systems produce different symptoms (see page 114 for more information on sensory systems and sensory processing disorder symptoms), but a child with sensory processing disorder typically finds the texture, smell, or even feel of food in their hands or mouth unpleasant. Eating is a negative experience for them, and they tend to be extremely picky about which foods they will accept.

In this chapter, you will learn about food sensitivity and sensory processing disorder, and how they can affect your child's ability to eat. In order to give you a full picture of how sensory processing works, we explain the brain's role in the process, how our bodies' specialized sensory systems work, and how problems within these specialized systems can affect how your child eats. A sensory processing disorder influences far more than your child's relationship with food, and the symptoms may be having a more noticeable impact on other areas of his life right now. We provide you with important information on the three main categories of sensory processing disorder and the symptoms your child might exhibit in all areas of his life, such as peer relationships, educational tasks, and community activities, so you are better able to assess whether he has a problem. You will also learn about feeding aversion (a condition in which a child fears putting things in his mouth) and how to recognize both the symptoms and causes. If you suspect your child has a sensory processing disorder or a feeding aversion, an occupational therapist will need to examine your child and consult with his pediatrician on a diagnosis. We'll explain what you can expect during the occupational therapist's evaluation and how she can help your child overcome his picky or problem eating. Finally, we offer several easy and effective strategies for teaching your child about food at home, as learning about food and growing accustomed to different textures, temperatures, smells, and flavors are crucial parts of helping your child manage his sensory processing issues.

FOOD-RELATED SENSORY PROCESSING DISORDER SYMPTOMS

Sensory processing disorder is a complex issue with symptoms that can affect many different areas of your child's life. However, since our focus is on picky and problem eating, let's begin with a list of sensory processing disorder symptoms that are directly related to feeding problems. If your child displays some or all of these symptoms, a sensory processing disorder is likely the culprit.

- Sensitivity to temperature of foods
- Sensitivity to food texture
- Sensitivity to smells
- Heightened awareness of flavor
- Lack of awareness of flavor
- Difficulty manipulating eating utensils
- Avoidance of touching foods
- Frequent spilling of both food and drinks unintentionally
- Chewing with mouth open
- Biting fingers and tongue while eating
- Dribbling food and drink down chin
- Dropping food on the floor unintentionally
- Constant fidgeting during the meal
- Variable attention during meals
- Frequent wiping of hands and mouth during eating
- Dislike of carbonated beverages

COULD YOUR CHILD HAVE JUST HAVE FOOD PREFERENCES INSTEAD OF A SENSORY PROCESSING DISORDER?

It's important to understand that we *all* have food preferences, meaning we all have certain foods that we dislike for some reason. For instance, some people don't like strawberries because they don't enjoy the sensation of eating a food with little seeds inside. Others may avoid crunchy peanut butter because they don't like how it looks. Minor food preferences such as these are normal and do not constitute picky or problem eating. They are simply a reflection of our personal tastes and do not interfere with our ability to eat a healthy, well-rounded diet. A sensory processing disorder is much more serious—it's a neurological condition that affects your child's ability to eat (or even touch) certain foods because of their sensory properties, and therefore affects your child's ability to meet and sustain his dietary needs. If your child is displaying a sensitivity to food that prevents him from eating or even touching a significant number of foods or entire food groups (as well as other symptoms listed below), he likely has a sensory processing disorder that requires evaluation and therapy from an occupational therapist who specializes in sensory processing disorders.

THE OCCUPATIONAL THERAPIST APPOINTMENT

An occupational therapist will evaluate your child's ability to process sensory information and determine if he has a sensory issue that is affecting his ability to eat. If he does, the occupational therapist will create a treatment program to help improve his tolerance of sensory input. She will assess your child's ability to use his hands and/or utensils during meals and select the best position for him to be in when he's eating. She will help you understand how your child interprets sensory input and work with you to develop a program to help your child enjoy his meals, not just endure them.

An occupational therapist has a diversified role within a feeding evaluation. The typical evaluation includes the following:

THE PHYSICAL EXAM

The therapist will evaluate your child's PROM (passive range of motion) and AROM (active range of motion). This means she will examine your child's neck, pelvis, and extremities to assess the mobility or limitations in movement of the joints. The therapist will be able to detect any musculoskeletal issues that may affect your child's positioning while eating. The therapist will also check the muscle tone of your child's chest and extremities to see if it is high, low, or fluctuates based on your child's position or motor action. Her findings will offer insight into your child's stamina for feeding and the best position for him to be in to eat a meal or snack. She will be able to offer recommendations for equipment adaptations for a feeding chair, utensils, cup, spoons, and so forth.

If your child has a diagnosed visual impairment or the therapist has concerns about his visual processing abilities, she may perform a visual-motor and visual-perceptual assessment. Vision issues can have a big impact on a child's ability to eat successfully. For instance, if your child has difficulty coordinating his eye movements, then he may have trouble perceiving an entire plate of food, grasping the foods with his hands, or using a spoon or cup for self-feeding.

THE PARENT INTERVIEW

During her interview with you, the occupational therapist will discuss your concerns about your child as well as the concerns any of the other health-care practitioners have expressed. She will also ask you questions about how and what your child eats. She will want to know the time of day (if any) that your child eats well. She will ask you to describe your typical mealtime process, from preparation to cleanup. The occupational therapist will ask you to describe the mealtime atmosphere as well. (Are meals typically rushed or calm? Smooth or chaotic? Noisy or quiet?) She'll ask you about how your kitchen is set up, what types of utensils are used, and how your child is seated during meals. (Is he in a high chair? Does he sit on a booster seat or a chair?) Then, with your help, the occupational therapist will put together a list of foods that your child likes and dislikes, and foods that vary from day to day.

THE FEEDING OBSERVATION

Like the speech therapist, the occupational therapist needs to observe your child during a meal for several reasons. First, she needs to assess firsthand the behaviors associated with the concerns you expressed during your interview with her. She will also want to assess your child's level of alertness before, during, and after a feeding. The occupational therapist will want to determine whether there are foods that increase or decrease your child's level of alertness. She will also be looking at your child's ability to pay attention during a meal, how your child reacts to distractions during a meal, and your child's ability to shift his attention during the meal from newly presented stimulation (i.e., discussing his day at school) to the agenda at hand, which is eating. She will observe whether there are foods that seem to increase or decrease your child's ability to pay attention. The therapist will also watch to see if your child displays any "true" defensiveness characteristics. A true defensiveness characteristic is an exaggerated and unpredictable reaction a child has to avoid sensory input, such as an illogical emotional outburst or severe self-injurious behavior.

THE SENSORY EVALUATION

One of the most important parts of the occupational therapist's exam is to evaluate how your child recognizes, processes, interprets, and organizes sensory information. This will help determine whether your child has a sensory processing disorder and if the established areas of concern are affecting his ability to eat.

There are many ways to gather information regarding your child's ability to process sensory information. The most effective methods are interviewing the parents and observing your child in his natural atmosphere as he plays, learns, and interacts with others. It's very important that the occupational therapist assess your child not only in isolation but in the context of his physical and social environment. It may take a few sessions for the therapist to gather the necessary information.

UNDERSTANDING SENSORY PROCESSING IN THE BRAIN

In order to understand how your child recognizes, processes, interprets, and organizes sensory information, you must understand what sensory processing is and the brain's role in the process.

Sensory processing is vital to our functioning because it's the foundation upon which develop all of our motor skills, social skills, and our capacity to learn and perform complex actions. The brain stem, which lies between the **spinal cord** and the higher centers of the brain, plays an integral role in processing sensory stimulation. The brain stem contains an important filtering system, which screens all incoming information to determine whether it should be noticed or disregarded. When there is a filtering problem, your child is overwhelmed by the information coming in, which can result in issues with motor coordination, difficulty relaying information among right/left hemispheres, difficulty maintaining attention, and regulation problems with breathing, heart rate, and digestion.

THE BRAIN STEM AND OUR SENSES

The brain stem also acts as a converging and relay station for sensations coming in through the different senses. It's designed to regulate sensory information we receive based on the demands of our environment and its current needs. The following mechanisms allow us to self-regulate:

- **Modulation:** The brain will turn neural switches on or off to regulate its activity and, subsequently, our activity level. It bases the regulation process on the task or activity we are doing. We need neural switches turned on to play a game of baseball and turned off to focus on reading a book.
- **Inhibition:** The brain will reduce connections between sensory intake and behavioral output when certain sensory information is not needed to perform a particular task. When your child is sitting in a classroom, her brain's sensory intake needs to inhibit the sounds coming from the humming fan so she can pay attention to the teacher. Her sensory system may become overstimulated if her brain does not block out unnecessary information.
- **Habituation:** When we become accustomed to familiar sensory messages, our brain automatically tunes them out. When you're in a car and put your seat belt on, the tautness of the seat belt may initially occupy your attention, but eventually you stop noticing it.
- **Facilitation:** The brain makes connections between sensory intake and behavioral output (what we sense and how we then react) by sending messages of displeasure (e.g., motion sickness) or pleasure (e.g., the calming feeling of a rocking chair). Facilitation lets us know when we need to stop activities

or will give us the "go ahead" signal for pleasurable activities.

OUR SPECIALIZED SENSORY SYSTEMS

We are all aware of the five senses—sight, hearing, taste, touch, and smell—but most people don't know that sensory processing also involves three additional specialized sensory systems, called the **vestibular, tactile,** and **proprioceptive systems.** These systems are known as the "power sensations" and influence how effectively we detect and make sense of vestibular (i.e., body movement in space), tactile (i.e., sensory input of touch) and proprioceptive (i.e., awareness of our body parts in space and their relation to one another) information. When this information is perceived, processed, and registered appropriately within the brain, your child will (for example):

- feel safe, secure, and comfortable in his own skin.
- play a reciprocal role in friendships (making eye contact, communicating, engaging in age-appropriate play, and so on).
- attend a birthday party for a friend at her house without feeling overwhelmed by the "newness" of the situation.
- direct and sustain his attention in the classroom even when multiple distractions are present.
- maneuver through an obstacle course on a scooter in PE class without loss of balance or feeling insecure (am I going to fall?).

- eat a nutritious meal from the four food groups without aversion.
- use his body to perform the myriad motor tasks we take for granted throughout a normal daily routine.

If your child has difficulties perceiving, processing, and registering the specialized sensory systems, he will become distracted by the multiple incoming sensory signals, which will greatly affect his performance in the above-mentioned tasks.

It's helpful to know what each specialized system does, because if your child has a sensory processing disorder, one or more of these systems may be affected.

THE VESTIBULAR SYSTEM

The vestibular system's receptors are located in the inner ear and sense movement of the head in all directions. The sensory input we receive through the vestibular system gives us subjective awareness of our body position in space (i.e., lying on your belly versus sitting in a bean bag chair versus standing on an uneven surface), communicates to us whether we are standing still or in motion, allows us to return to midline if our equilibrium is challenged (i.e., righting yourself as you trip), and allows for stabilization of our eyes during head movement (i.e., keeping eyes stabilized while spinning around in circles). It also affects muscle tone, posture, and eye movements (i.e., reading a newspaper or focusing your eyes on the taillights of the car ahead of you in a snowstorm, etc.), and perceptual abilities (i.e., the spatial relationships between objects such as pouring milk into a glass).

Here's an example of the importance of the vestibular processing system and its relationship to feeding. Five-year-old Ben tended to use his chair at the dinner table like the jungle gym at school, maneuvering all around it. This behavior was really distracting to Ben's parents and siblings, but every time they physically stopped him (he didn't respond to verbal commands), Ben had a meltdown.

After evaluating the child, the occupational therapist determined that Ben demonstrated characteristics suggestive of a sensory processing disorder. Maneuvering all around the chair at mealtime gave Ben an awareness of his body in space, which he needed for the oral motor and postural demands necessary for eating. It was also a way to calm himself during meals because the feeding environment was very loud and chaotic.

The therapist recommended that a footstool with foot straps be placed under Ben's feet to help him feel "grounded" and a specialized therapy cushion be placed on his chair. This would allow him to seek the input he needed during a meal in a controlled manner. She also suggested that Ben's parents limit distractions at mealtime and created a customized program of vestibular and proprioceptive input (movement activities coupled with gross motor activities) for Ben to engage in prior to meals. This allowed Ben to enter the mealtime atmosphere with improved awareness of his body position in space and allow his internal "sensory framework" to be calm, organized, and balanced.

THE PROPRIOCEPTIVE SYSTEM

The proprioceptive system has its receptors in muscles, tendons, and joints. Sensory information from this system is created by the contraction and stretching of muscles and by the bending and straightening, pulling and compression of joints between bones. The most effective means for feedback of proprioceptive information occurs when resistance is present during muscle contraction (see Sara's story below for an example of this concept). This information is constantly being sent to the brain to tell us about the body's position in space and offer us awareness about our body parts in space. When we have adequate proprioceptive processing, our brain has a "map" of all our body parts and their current function without relying on our conscious attention.

Here is an example that illustrates the impact proprioceptive input has on the success of a child drinking from a cup. Six-year-old Sara has sensory processing issues, and her parents bring her to see a speech therapist. One of her parents' complaints is that their daughter will only drink from a pink, no-spill, ten-ounce cup at school. They have tried numerous cups, and this is the only one Sara will accept. After the speech therapist assessed Sara using the cup, she explained to the parents that this particular cup has a no-spill valve. This valve creates a vacuum, which offers Sara resistance while drinking. (Remember: the most effective means for feedback of proprioceptive information occurs when resistance is present during muscle contraction.) This resistance provides Sara with proprioceptive input, which serves as a calming and organizing force. By understanding Sara's proprioceptive needs as related to the skill of cup drinking, we can understand why she prefers the no-spill cup. Now her parents and therapist are better equipped to assist her in transitioning to an open-face cup.

THE TACTILE SYSTEM

The tactile system has a profound influence on our ability to learn. It houses touch receptors located just under the skin, which define our body boundaries and differentiate **light touch** from **pressure touch**. Light touch is a diffuse sensation that spreads quickly throughout the body. We are born with this system intact. It's responsible for alerting the nervous system to be wary of possible danger and draws our attention to either approaching the tactile input or avoiding it entirely. Pressure touch receptors are located deeper under the skin's surface and have a slow response time. They are responsible for calming the nervous system and allowing us to tolerate approaching touch from others. They also provide a localized discriminating sensation, which enables us to tell shapes, textures, and sizes of handheld objects without looking at them, also known as **stereognosis**. This system matures after birth.

The tactile system is crucial to our ability to function on a daily basis, and problems within this system are physically, mentally, and emotionally exhausting, especially for a child with tactile processing issues. Imagine how a toddler at a birthday party would feel if he couldn't touch vanilla ice cream with candy sprinkles because the texture of the sprinkles mixed with the texture of the ice cream was nauseating to him. Or imagine being overly sensitive to any type of touch and having to remain in a defensive mode, always on alert to the possibility of an unpleasant sensation. Not fun.

The tactile system is the one system that is directly related to feeding difficulties. Children with tactile processing issues often have unusual, limited food preferences. Many prefer bland, textureless foods, and will tolerate eating only a few favorite foods: chips, fast-food chicken nuggets, and chocolate milk, for example. This is because children with tactile sensory problems are often comfortable with the sensory properties of only particular foods (i.e., the appearance, smell, taste, and texture of the food). If a child is uncomfortable with the sensory properties of a food, he won't even touch it with his hand, let alone try to eat it.

DID YOU KNOW?

Many children with sensory processing disorder become increasingly selective about what they eat as they grow and mature. They find comfort and emotional well-being in seeking out predictable foods that are familiar to them. This is their way of protecting themselves from being overwhelmed by the sensory properties of "new" foods.

SENSORY PROCESSING DISORDER

As you now know, sensory processing refers to our ability to recognize sensory input, interpret and process this information, organize the input, and make a meaningful response. For most people, this process is automatic. Children who have a sensory processing disorder, however, don't experience this process in the same way. A sensory processing disorder affects the way a child's brain interprets the information they take in and also how they act on that information.

A sensory processing disorder not only affects your child's ability to eat, it also has an impact on important skills and preparatory factors that are directly related to eating. For instance, if your child has a sensory processing issue, it may affect his motor coordination, which he needs to use utensils effectively. It may prevent your child from participating in and tolerating the mealtime experience, as we saw with Ben on page 116. It may affect your child's tolerance of smells from foods. It may also affect your child's tolerance for pain and noise, and myriad other things. In order to help you determine whether your child may be suffering from a sensory processing disorder, we discuss below the three main categories—sensory modulation, sensory discrimination, and sensory-based motor disorder—and offer you a list of typical symptoms from all areas of life that your child might exhibit.

When the occupational therapist evaluates your child's sensory processing abilities, she will gauge whether they fall within one or more of these categories.

DID YOU KNOW?

We've all experienced "sensory overload" and become stressed to the point that we can no longer focus. Children with a sensory processing disorder struggle with this feeling on a daily basis, and sometimes teachers or parents will observe "behavioral outbursts." For example, a teacher reported that a child with sensory processing disorder began banging his crayon box against his head in the middle of the holiday class party. When asked about the outburst, the teacher said it occurred "out of the blue," with no warning. Upon assessing the situation, we discovered that there was too much sensory stimulation present for this student and he experienced "sensory overload." He didn't have an efficient internal mechanism in place to cope with the excess sensory stimulation, so he looked externally for a way to calm himself. Now, this does not mean that the child should be excluded from the class parties—his parents and teachers just need to come up with strategies to help him during times when excess sensory stimulation is present (like a noisy holiday party or school assembly). Strategies could include having the child help the teacher set up for the party and providing him with "outlets" to calm himself during the party, such as fidget toys that he can manipulate with his hands. This will enable him to actively participate with his peers in the next party, not just endure the party. This example shows why it's so important that "behavioral outbursts" are thoroughly assessed to determine whether a child is experiencing sensory overload or simply acting out. If a child is experiencing sensory overload, then outbursts of this kind are his way of communicating that he needs external help to regulate his sensory system.

SENSORY MODULATION DISORDER

There are several types of attributes that indicate a child has a sensory modulation disorder. He may be:

- Underresponsive (demonstrates a decreased sensitivity to sensory input)
- Overresponsive (demonstrates increased sensitivity to sensory input)
- A sensory seeker (has an innate desire for more stimulation and never seems to be fulfilled by the amount or intensity of the stimulation)
- A sensory fluctuator (fluctuates between underresponsiveness and overresponsiveness)

THE UNDERRESPONSIVE CHILD

Some children are underresponsive to sensory input or demonstrate a decreased sensitivity to sensory input. Their nervous systems do not always recognize the sensory information that is coming in to the brain. As a result, they appear to have an almost insatiable desire for sensory stimulation. They seek out constant stimulation or more intense or prolonged sensory experiences, often by taking part in extreme activities or moving constantly. Underresponsive kids often exhibit the following characteristics:

- They disregard touch from objects or people unless it is intense.
- They are unaware of having a messy face after eating an ice cream cone, messy hands after playing in the mud, or wet socks after playing in the snow.

- They have minimal response to painful stimuli, such as booster shots or broken bones.
- They lack the initiative to participate in movement experiences.
- They have poor body awareness, which interferes with dressing, feeding, writing, and playing.
- They have a difficult time responding quickly to objects approaching them, such as a ball toss.
- They don't seem to respond to ordinary sounds, soft voices, and whispers.

Mealtime Snapshot

If your child is underresponsive, he may appear unaware of or oblivious to the mealtime experience, even in highly stimulating environments like a family holiday gathering. He may have a difficult time differentiating among the tastes, temperatures, textures, and smells of foods. In fact, if you were to ask, he may describe most foods as tasting pretty much the same. Because of this, your child may submerge his food in spicy or hot condiments to help get a sense of how the food tastes. He may also have a difficult time identifying the sensation of feeling full, which can result in portion control issues because he doesn't know when to stop eating.

THE OVERRESPONSIVE CHILD

Other children with a sensory processing disorder are overresponsive to sensory input. Their nervous systems feel sensation too easily or too intensely, and they feel as if they are being constantly bombarded with information. They often describe this feeling of bombardment as fireworks going off around them without any predictability. Consequently, these children often have a "fight or flight" response to a particular sensory input or a combination of sensory stimuli. Overresponsive kids often display the following characteristics:

- They may try to avoid or minimize sensations, by avoiding being touched or being very particular about clothing and footwear.
- They tend to be very picky eaters and/or overly sensitive to food smells.
- They prefer long sleeves and pants to eliminate skin exposure or prefer short sleeves and pants so that the clothing does not rub against the skin.
- They isolate themselves from playground activities, avoid physical activities, and are very uncomfortable in highly distractible environments, such as a birthday party.
- They are sensitive to lights and may become nauseated by moving objects or people.
- They are uncomfortable with loud noises, high-pitched noises, or sudden, unexpected noises.

Mealtime Snapshot

If your child is overresponsive, he may be extremely picky about the foods he will eat and overly sensitive to the smells of food. He may have a tendency to avoid meals because the mealtime atmosphere is overwhelming to him. Your child may not appear to have much of an appetite, and he may avoid touching or manipulating food. This is a significant issue, because if your child is uncomfortable manipulating food, he will not learn about the properties of food and won't establish a "sensory memory" of what foods are like for when he encounters them in the future. And, of course, if your child is uncomfortable manipulating food in his hands, he certainly won't be eating it.

THE SENSORY SEEKER

The sensory seeker is the child who loves sensory stimulation so much that he can never get enough. His nervous system requires a huge amount and intensity of stimulation and the child enjoys every minute of it. This child is viewed by others as a risk taker and as a result is often described by others as a troublemaker. Sensory-seeking children often exhibit the following characteristics:

- They seem to always be touching and feeling objects, bumping into people or objects, and like to be close to people.
- They enjoy being involved in messy experiences for long periods of time.
- They love powerful movement experiences (such as hanging upside down on the monkey bars or spinning round and round on a scooter board).
- They love physical activity, especially jumping and diving.

- They like being close to bright lights and strobe lights.
- They like loud noises and commotion and see unexpected noises as "fun."

Mealtime Snapshot

Your child may love to explore the sensory properties of food but have a difficult time transitioning from that to another task, such as doing his homework, without having a meltdown. He may become "lost" in the act of eating and spend a great deal of time eating in an effort to satisfy his sensory needs. Much like the underresponsive child, your sensory seeker may eat and eat and eat, disregarding his sensation of feeling full. In fact, he may use food as a comfort measure.

THE SENSORY FLUCTUATOR

A child who fluctuates between underresponsiveness and overresponsiveness is extremely difficult to understand. There never seems to be a pattern to help us predict the sensory stimulation he seeks or avoids. One day the child may crave intense movement experiences, such as spinning around and around on a scooter board, and the next day he may avoid it completely. This child is exhausting to parent and to teach because his sensory disposition varies from day to day and hour to hour. The parents of a sensory fluctuator struggle not only with how to help their child but with understanding what the appropriate intervention for their child should be at a given moment in time on a daily basis.

Mealtime Snapshot

If your child fluctuates between underresponsiveness and overresponsiveness, his mealtime behavior may be very hard to predict from one meal to the next. He likely exhibits a mixture of mealtime/feeding behaviors from both the under-responsive and overresponsive categories above.

SENSORY DISCRIMINATION DISORDER

A child with sensory discrimination disorder processes sensory input inefficiently and is unable to make meaningful responses in the world around him. The problem lies in the "intake" of sensory information, and it directly affects a child's ability to learn from, interact with, and explore the environment. Children with sensory discrimination disorder often display the following characteristics:

- They have difficulty identifying familiar objects with their eyes closed.
- They are unable to distinguish between similar items such as a brush and a comb.
- They have difficulty in tactile perception or recognizing the physical properties of an object or food (i.e., texture, form, temperature).
- They have difficulty dressing, grooming, eating, and performing hygiene tasks.
- They have difficulty knowing where their bodies are in space as they relate to people and objects.
- They have trouble stringing beads, following a

pattern to complete a block design, and understanding directional concepts.

- They have difficulty spacing letters and orienting words and sentences on a line.
- They have difficulty explaining their thoughts to others, either verbally or in written format.
- They have difficulty tracking a sound in the room and trouble recognizing differences in sounds, words, phrases, and sentences.
- They have trouble with verbal problem solving and organizing pieces of information into a comprehensive story.

Mealtime Snapshot

Your child may have a difficult time discriminating among various sensory input as it relates to the taste, temperature, texture, and smell of foods. For example, your child may not be able to identify the visual differences between an apple and a tomato, the difference between the smell of a lemon and the smell of an orange, the difference between a Cheerio and a cracker as he manipulates them in his hand, or the temperature difference between ice cream and warm apple crisp as he explores these vastly different food properties with his mouth. This will ultimately affect his ability to create an accurate memory of food that he can call upon when he encounters these foods in the future.

SENSORY-BASED MOTOR DISORDERS

There are two sensory-based motor disorders that your child

may have: postural disorder and dyspraxia. Children with a postural disorder often exhibit:

- Difficulty coordinating use of both sides of the body as needed to ride a bike, skip, and play sports.
- Difficulty maintaining equilibrium while standing still (freeze tag is very difficult for these children).
- Poor control of eye movements, which affects their depth perception and crossing midline skills, or the ability to reach across the body with an arm to retrieve an object.

Children with dyspraxia have trouble initiating, planning, and carrying out new motor skills. These kids have particular difficulty with forming a goal or idea. Children with dyspraxia often display the following characteristics:

- They are clumsy, awkward, and accident prone, which unfortunately leads to low self-esteem.
- Their muscles are weak and they fatigue easily.
- They have poor gross/fine motor control and poor eye-hand coordination.
- They have difficulty using both hands/feet together in play or in an alternating manner.
- They struggle with handwriting, drawing, or visual reproduction tasks and may try to compensate with an overreliance on language.
- They may prefer noncompetitive games with peers over competitive sports. They also tend to play the

role of the "coach" or "referee" in neighborhood or playground games to avoid active participation.
- They may try to mask their motor planning problems by acting like a "class clown" or avoiding new group activities.

Mealtime Snapshot

If your child has a sensory-based motor disorder, he may use up all of his energy on postural control, draining him of the stamina he needs to complete a meal. He may have a difficult time using utensils and may often revert to using his hands. Your child may have a difficult time with the fine-motor coordination needed for sequencing instructions of a recipe (i.e., folding the tortilla to make an enchilada) and following mealtime directions, such as grabbing a blue basket of rolls and passing it to his brother.

DID YOU KNOW?

Children with a sensory processing disorder may become distracted by the tags in their clothes, the unpredictability of other children, the "tickling" of hair on their ears, the buzzing of the lighting units in the classroom, the sound level in gym class, smells in the cafeteria, rearrangement of the classroom after a holiday break, and subtle changes in planned meals (i.e., chicken sandwiches instead of chicken tacos for dinner). This can prompt them to seek regular, familiar routines, which helps them to feel safe, comfortable, and in control of the world around them.

GENERAL SENSORY PROCESSING DISORDER SYMPTOMS

As we mentioned earlier, sensory processing disorder affects children in many different ways. Our focus in this chapter is on sensory processing disorder and its influence on feeding, but it's important to remember that if your child has feeding difficulties, more than one sensory system is typically involved. Below is a description of symptoms in relation to each of the five senses, which will help you more easily identify attributes in your child and better understand the complexity of the problem:

AUDITORY

If your child is sensitive to auditory stimulation, he may be more successful eating his meals in a setting that offers few distractions. At home you might offer your child meals at the kitchen table with a few overhead lights on, the television and radio turned off, and the phone taken off the hook. At school the ideal spot for eating would be in the quietest corner of the cafeteria. A noisy, busy restaurant or school cafeteria can easily become a negative experience for your child, as the high level of distraction may render him unable to focus on his meal.

Alternatively, if your child is hyporesponsive to auditory stimulation, he may seem oblivious to what is going on around him or demonstrate variable attention or limited attention to his meal, which means it may take him a long time to finish a meal. This is especially a problem for families with a fast-paced lifestyle as well as at school, where lunch periods are limited. Your child may seem to eat better amid a lot of chaos and noise, or he may tend to isolate himself during meals because the noise is so overwhelming that he simply can't even try to eat, even if he is hungry.

VISUAL

The very task of eating can be overwhelming to a visually sensitive child. If your child is sensitive to visual stimulation, he may become overwhelmed by the appearance of a table cluttered with serving bowls, plates, dishes, silverware, and glasses. He may be more comfortable entering the mealtime experience with fewer visual distractions. Try using green-colored place mats (the color green has a calming effect) with only the glasses and silverware set at each place setting. Place the serving bowls, napkins, and plates on the counter and have your child grab his plate and scoop out food onto his plate himself. Your child should be the first person to serve himself so when he sits at the table, the appearance of the table will still be pretty uniform. It's important to remember that the appearance of your child's plate may also be overwhelming to him if food portions are too large or there are too many food choices on the plate. Try giving your child a divided plate, which will provide you with a visual guide for serving sizes, or, if your child can serve himself, allow him control over how food is organized on his plate.

Some children are also sensitive to the appearance of food items. Your child may dislike certain colors or combinations of colors when it comes to food and refuse to eat meals based solely on their visual presentation.

Your child may also seek out colors to help him organize the

visual information he needs to eat meals. For exa
give your child a black place mat and a white tod
his food, it may not only help him locate his plate on the table but also allow him to identify and manipulate the foods on his plate through contrasting colors (i.e., green peas versus orange slices on the white plate). You could also try using colored spoons and forks with a white plate to help improve your child's accuracy in scooping or poking the food with his utensils. A bright red cup instead of a clear glass may help your child grasp his cup more successfully.

Many visually sensitive children are sensitive to bright lights or fluorescent lighting often used in restaurants and schools. It's also not uncommon for them to "zone out" on particular objects during meals. This is actually a strategy these kids use to calm themselves in stressful situations, as it helps them separate themselves from visual stimulation that they find overwhelming.

TASTE/SMELL

If your child is sensitive to tastes he will avoid those that are unpleasant to him at meals and, in extreme cases, he will refuse the remainder of a meal if he perceives a taste as unpleasant. Your child may be a "super taster" and seek strong flavors of food. He may prefer hot or spicy seasoning on his food or eat a food like a lemon without any noticeable reaction to the very sour flavor. Or your child may be extremely sensitive to taste, especially the aftertaste of food or drinks. Medications may be extremely noxious for him. Your child may be hypersensitive to some odors and may even become nauseated to the point of vomiting. He may refuse to enter the kitchen or sit at the table if he smells an odor that is unpleasant to him. Alternatively, your child may not seem to notice strong odors at all, or he may seek out strong odors and smell every bite of food before eating it and/or smell nonfood items.

TOUCH

If your child is sensitive to touch, he may avoid touching food with his hands and pull his hands away from the plate when you place it in front of him. He may run away from a food he views as unpleasant or remove the food from his plate with a utensil so that he does not come in contact with it. If he encounters a texture he perceives as unpleasant, he may become distressed if he does not have a napkin or wet washcloth beside his plate at meals. He may gag when touching food or gag easily while eating. Your child may consistently "play" with or explore his food as a way to become engaged in the mealtime experience. He may seem unaware of the differences in food properties and act as though all food tastes the same.

In addition to the impact on the senses while your child is eating, sensory problems can also affect your child's coordination of body movement, balance, attention, behavior, social skills, and speech language development. We recommend Carol Stock Kranowitz's *The Out-of-Sync Child: Recognizing and Coping with Sensory Processing Disorder* for a more in-depth look at sensory processing disorder and all its symptoms. It's an excellent resource for parents of a child with sensory processing disorder.

DIAGNOSING SENSORY PROCESSING DISORDER

The occupational therapist cannot diagnose your child with a sensory processing disorder. Her role is to compile the information necessary for a diagnosis and share it with your child's pediatrician. It's important that the occupational therapist be knowledgeable and trained in the area of sensory processing disorders in order to properly assess your child and interpret the findings of each piece of the evaluation. The pediatrician will then diagnose your child based on the information the therapist provides. In order to gather the necessary information on your child, the occupational therapist may use a sensory processing standardized tool or an observational checklist to assist in the evaluation process.

FEEDING AVERSION

"How did we get to the point where a good day is determined by whether or not my child eats more than a few bites of food?" says Karen, the mother of eight-year-old Lisa. Sound familiar? This is the type of frustration we often hear voiced by parents of children with feeding aversion, also known as **oral defensiveness.** A child with feeding aversion is extremely apprehensive about and commonly fears any interaction having to do with his mouth. She fears that this interaction will produce discomfort and/or pain, often resulting in a negative response to some or all food tastes, smells, and textures. A child with feeding aversion simply cannot enjoy eating.

Feeding aversion is a complex problem. It can be caused by a sensory processing disorder as well as by previous medical procedures, such as placement of a feeding tube. Fortunately, there are patterns that we can identify to help us locate the root cause of feeding aversion in individual children. In order to fully understand your child's feeding aversion, the occupational therapist will need key information from you regarding your child's birth history, a report of the first days of feeding after your child was born, and a report of the feeding successes and difficulties in the first few year(s) of her life. It is crucial to gather the information from the newborn stage because breast- or bottle-feeding lays the foundation for future feeding skills.

HAS YOUR CHILD MASTERED THE SUCK/SWALLOW/BREATHE SEQUENCE?

During feeding, an infant must learn to coordinate three separate acts—sucking, swallowing, and breathing, or the "suck/swallow/breathe sequence"—to be able to eat successfully. This skill is vital to master, as it affects eating both now and in the future. All other feeding skills are built upon this sequence. Problems mastering this stage of eating can spiral into additional feeding and health problems, including aspiration. (An infant's airway is very close to the esophagus, and sometimes small or large amounts of liquid can travel down between the vocal cords into the airway. This is called aspiration.) Aspiration can make an infant very ill. He may develop frequent colds, congestion, unexplained fevers, or aspiration pneumonia. In its most severe form, aspiration can be fatal. In order to make a proper assessment of your child, the occupational therapist will need to know the following:

- Did your child feel safe eating as an infant? Infants are excellent communicators, and they are able to tell us if they are content while they are feeding or if they are having difficulties. All we need to do is observe their "baby responses" during feedings, such as facial gestures, color changes, body movements, and state changes (i.e., calm state to irritable state). If your child had difficulty feeding as an infant, he may have cried, turned his head, grimaced, and/or arched his back to escape the nipple. Frequent coughing, choking, or gagging during feedings are also indicators that a child is having difficulty with feeding. A baby who has loud audible swallows and then panting (recovery breathing) or formula spilling out of his mouth while feeding may have been communicating to you that the nipple flow rate was too fast. All of these responses indicate that your child may have felt *unsafe* eating as an infant.
- Did you have difficulty bottle- or breast-feeding? For instance, did your child have a problem latching on to the breast or did liquid pour out of her mouth during bottle feedings?
- Did liquid spill from his mouth?
- Were feedings excessively long in duration? Did your baby sound gurgly or gulpy while feeding?
- Did your baby have any coughing spells or color change while feeding? If so, the liquid may actually

have been going down the wrong way toward the airway, which indicates possible laryngeal penetration and/or aspiration.

If you answered "yes" to these questions, your child may have had difficulty mastering the suck/swallow/breathe sequence, which would affect his mastery of the foundational oral-motor skills necessary for feeding. Remember, if your child does not have the foundation skills of the suck/swallow/breathe sequence and the correct tongue configuration for feeding, then he will have difficulty advancing to more difficult oral motor tasks as he grows, such as clearing food from a spoon, moving the tongue correctly to move thicker-consistency food (puree) around in the mouth, and coordinating controlled tongue movements that are necessary to move food over to the teeth to chew. A child who has had previous difficulties with bottle- or breast-feeding, such as feeling unsafe and/or overwhelmed with the flow of milk during breast- or bottle-feeding, will create a "memory" of feeding as being unpleasant, and this memory could potentially lead to a feeding aversion.

HAS YOUR CHILD HAD TROUBLE WITH FOOD TRANSITIONS?

Some children have difficulty transitioning from formula or breast milk to baby food or from baby food to table food. There are several reasons for this. Some children struggle with eating because of an oral motor problem, such as having difficulty moving the muscles of their lips, cheeks, and tongue in a coordinated manner to bite, chew, and swallow food safely. Other children have oral sensory issues in which they tend to be overresponsive, underresponsive, or variable in interpreting the sensory properties of foods in their mouths. Some children have both oral motor and sensory issues that cause transition problems. These types of problems can cause further difficulties when it comes to controlling food or liquid in the mouth. Symptoms of food transition problems include watery eyes, coughing, gagging, choking, and spitting food out of the mouth. Children who have trouble with food transitions feel overwhelmingly unsafe and start avoiding the act of eating, which can lead to the development of food aversion.

TEACHING YOUR CHILD ABOUT FOOD

In this fast-paced age, having a "family meal" together is no longer the norm. Many families rely on both the mother and the father for income, and the children are often involved in after-school activities. Unfortunately, many of these activities typically run during or past the dinnertime meal hour, which has a big impact on family mealtimes. But sitting at the dinner table as a family and taking the time to teach your child about different foods is a key part of broadening his food horizons. If your child is exposed to the same few foods every day, he won't learn how to manage the complex sensory information he needs to eat difficult foods, such as raw vegetables, hard-to-chew meats, or slippery fruits.

Every exposure your child has to a variety of foods will help improve his acceptance of the taste, texture, aroma, and appearance of the foods you offer at meals. Here are some activities you can do with your child at home to teach him about the properties of food. Make sure to discuss the properties of the foods you're using with each activity.

- Encourage your child to open the lids of containers or the packages of food, or grab a kiwi or some asparagus out of the crisper for you, so he can become accustomed to the smell, appearance, and texture of the food. Talk about the properties of the food before you begin handling or tasting it.
- Show your child how fun it can be to stir food, squash it, smell it, pour it into different containers, and dump it out again. If your child is uncomfortable having direct contact with the food, that's OK. Have him use nonlatex gloves, cover his hands in plastic wrap, or use paintbrushes or wooden play utensils to explore the food.
- Sit down at the table and play with food—squish it, wiggle it, poke it, finger paint with the food to make animal or people pictures, let your child break it open with his hands. Let your child make a mess with the food, even if he puts it on his face or body, or in his hair. Encourage any kind of interaction he has with food.
- Create a food chart out of poster board to categorize food properties with the following descriptors: crunchy, soft, wet, flaky, smooth, slimy, tough,

rough, bumpy, squishy, tart, and sweet. Make it a family activity, and have each family member provide input. You could use the chart at each meal or designate a certain meal each day to use it.

- With a pair of scissors, cut various colors of felt into the shapes of different foods and pretend to feed them to stuffed animals or dolls with your child.
- Purchase a food coloring book and color in foods together.
- Use foods as a coloring modality. For example, use a pretzel stick and melted cheese to draw a mouse, or use an Oreo cookie and frosting to draw the cookie monster.
- Take foods and make a picture of a person (i.e., vanilla wafers for eyes, licorice strings for hair, M&M's for eyes, a jelly bean for a nose, Bugles for fingers, and pretzel sticks for arms and legs).
- Take your child to the grocery store and hand him your grocery list. Enlist his help in finding some or all of the foods and placing them in the cart. This is an invaluable experience and a great way for you to expose him to many different foods at one time.
- Play with toy foods. Playing restaurant, going on a pretend picnic, and having a princess tea party can be a lot of fun. Children enjoy feeding toy food to puppets. You can follow up the activity with re-creating your evening meal with real foods.
- Use cookie cutters to cut food into different shapes.

- Show your child how foods pull apart and how to crush them up.
- Welcome little hands into the kitchen. Cook meals with your child, let him gather the ingredients and discuss the food properties, let him measure the foods, let him smell the foods, watch cooking shows with him, or look through kid-friendly cookbooks with your child for fun recipes to follow.

If it is determined that your child has a sensory processing disorder that is affecting his eating, you will work with both the occupational therapist and the speech therapist (see chapter 3 for more information on the speech therapist's role in food chaining) to develop a customized program to help your child recognize, understand, and actively explore the sensory properties of foods.

CHAPTER 5

How Can I Stop the Mealtime Battles and Other Negative Behaviors?

The Behavioral Evaluation

Jenny, mother of three-year-old twins Kylie and Kaylie, has been having feeding troubles with her kids ever since she tried to transition them to baby food at four months of age. The family had just moved to a new town, and the isolation was especially hard on Jenny, who had no help with her babies. Kylie and Kaylie were not sleeping well, and neither was Jenny. She decided to start spoon-feeding the babies because everyone told her that might help them sleep better. They hated it. Kylie gagged, and Kaylie didn't know what to do with the cereal. She spit it right back out of her mouth. Jenny persisted, but the girls never seemed to get the hang of spoon-feeding. A few months later, at six months, she offered them turkey bacon baby food, which they ate with no problem. However, when she tried to give them other baby foods, the girls wouldn't eat them. For months, Kylie and Kaylie only ate turkey bacon baby food and took their bottles. When they were close to a year old, Jenny started offering table food. Every time she offered something new, the girls cried and turned away or gagged. Then they even stopped wanting the turkey bacon baby food. Jenny's mother offered them bites of pancake one day, and they liked that. But after that seemingly successful meal they again started showing the same pattern. They only wanted pancakes. They ate pancakes for months. This continued until eventually Jenny was able to get them to accept fast-food french fries and animal crackers. Now meals are more and more of a struggle. Kaylie has started to show some "bad" mealtime behaviors. She screams and cries at every meal. She won't sit in her chair. She won't come to the table and screams the whole time if she is forced. Kylie, on the other hand, doesn't fuss at all. She just pushes food away and rejects it. She seems genuinely upset by new food. Jenny is at the end of her rope because nothing she does is helping. She dreads mealtimes.

JUST AS YOU need to identify any medical, physical, and sensory issues that may be contributing to your child's feeding problems before starting to food chain, so, too, do you need to understand behaviors that may be playing a role.

You may be feeling helplessness and despair over your children's behavior. "I've tried everything, but I don't know how to make things better," says Sally, the parent of a seven-year-old. Some parents feel guilty because they believe they are to blame for their children's negative behaviors. Still others become angry and defensive because they think others blame them for how their child acts. These are all normal responses and nothing to feel ashamed about. However, know that your child's feeding problems and her behavior are not your fault. The professionals who work with picky and problem eaters know all too well that young kids can be master manipulators and know exactly which buttons to push to get their parents to react. In this chapter, we tackle the negative behaviors most commonly seen at the table and discuss what may be prompting your child to act this way. You'll learn how to use positive reinforcement to encourage good behavior in your child and strategies for diffusing bad mealtime behaviors when they occur. We also discuss the importance of a behavioral psychologist on a feeding team and the role he plays in the process, and debunk the stereotypes that prevent many people from reaching out to a behavioral psychologist for help.

YOUR CHILD'S NEGATIVE BEHAVIOR SPEAKS VOLUMES

We believe that a child's negative behavior holds the key to understanding why she is having feeding problems. Your child is behaving in certain ways because she's trying to *tell* you something. By learning to interpret your child's behavior, you can figure out where the feeding process is breaking down for her. If your child refuses to come to the table, she may not be able to tolerate the appearance of a full table or the aromas of different foods combined. If your child spits food out, she may not be able to handle the sensations inside her mouth during chewing. It's true that some children use negative behavior at meals to get their parents' attention, but more often negative mealtime behavior indicates an underlying sensory issue with food. As was the case with Kylie and Kaylie, serious behaviors can develop from sensory issues with food. Abnormal meals become the norm, and the stress level in your home can sky-rocket. These negative behaviors can be changed, and this chapter offers you the tools to help make it happen. Common negative mealtime behaviors include:

- Refusing to come to the table
- Leaving the table during the meal
- Crying when food is presented
- Spitting food out
- Throwing food
- Disrupting others who are trying to eat
- Being unable to focus on meals

DID YOU KNOW?

Research shows that only 12 percent of feeding disorders are purely behavioral in nature. So if your child is a picky or problem eater, it is very likely that she suffers from one or more of the conditions that we describe in the previous four chapters.

SHOULD YOU SEE A BEHAVIORAL PSYCHOLOGIST?

This chapter will provide strategies for handling your child's negative mealtime behaviors. However, if your child is strong-willed or acts out frequently both at meals and outside of meals, a behavioral psychologist can give valuable insight into your child's behavior and help you create and implement strategies for lasting change. There are also situations where a feeding problem is just one symptom of a larger problem, such as a child's reaction to her parents' divorce or a choking incident that traumatized her. Sometimes a feeding problem can indicate a control issue between a child and her parents, where she is manipulating her parents with her food intake. Only a trained behavioral psychologist is qualified to address these types of issues and help your child get back on track. If your child's behavior is significantly affecting her nutritional status, she is exhibiting phobic reactions to new foods (such as a panicked look on her face when offered a new food or shaky hands when trying a new food), her behavior appears out of control, or continues to worsen over time, we strongly suggest that you seek out help from a behavioral psychologist.

We understand that sometimes even the mere mention of a psychologist in relation to your child or your family can be unsettling. There is an unfortunate stigma attached to those who work in the mental health community, and many people feel that seeing a psychologist automatically means something is wrong with them. This is simply not true. A behavioral psychologist's job is to provide important pieces of the puzzle that is your child's feeding disorder, in the same way that the pediatrician, dietitian, speech therapist, and occupational therapist do.

When you choose to work with a psychologist, you are choosing to work with a professional who can help improve the health and happiness of your family. You are choosing to work with someone who can give your child the tools she needs to be successful in life. As parents, that's all we really want for our kids.

THE BEHAVIORAL PSYCHOLOGIST APPOINTMENT

Sometimes a behavioral psychologist will already be part of a feeding team, but that's not always the case. If you need to find one on your own, ask one or more of the members of your feeding team to recommend a psychologist who has experience treating children with feeding disorders. It's very important that the psychologist you choose does have some degree of experience working with picky or problem eaters, and the more experience he has, the better. Or, you can ask your friends or your child's teachers for recommendations.

Once you've gotten the contact information for a behavioral psychologist you'd like to try, we suggest you briefly interview him by phone or face to face. Ask a few questions. Listen to your feelings and trust your intuition. Don't hesitate to change your mind and seek another psychologist if you don't feel satisfied. It's important that the psychologist you choose be someone both you and your child feel comfortable and safe with.

Here are some questions to ask during your interview:

- What type of license do you have?
- What are your credentials and/or certifications?
- Can you tell me about your experience with children who have had feeding disorders?
- How many kids with feeding disorders have you treated?
- Are you up-to-date on current information on feeding disorders?
- What type of therapy do you practice?
- How long are your sessions?
- If you are away, do you have coverage?
- Do you take my insurance?

There is no one way for a behavioral psychologist to evaluate a child. His approach will depend largely on the nature of your child's problems. The psychologist may see your child in his office or he may go to your child's school or your home to observe her behavior. If she's having problems in school, the psychologist may recommend she take standardized tests to determine her IQ and whether she's where she should be developmentally. Your child may have more than just a feeding problem to address, such as sleep issues, anxiety, or her relationship with you or your partner, so the evaluation could take several sessions instead of one. The psychologist will likely also want to meet with your entire family, both to ask questions and to help mediate any problems your child is having with other family members. As we mentioned earlier, he will also help keep the flow of communication strong between your family and the feeding team during your child's food-chaining program.

A large part of the behavioral psychologist's job is to evaluate the strategies you use to handle your child's behavior. It's critical for him to determine whether your strategies and your child's learning style are a good fit. That's not to say that there's anything *wrong* with your strategies. It just means that sometimes certain aspects of a parenting style just don't work well with the personality or learning style of a child. Even small adjustments can go a long way toward improving your child's feeding problem. He may do this by coming to your home to observe a meal or by viewing a videotape you make of a meal with your child.

Once the psychologist has assessed how your child is best able to learn, he will consult with her feeding team on the most effective ways to teach your child about food. He will be able to give you clear instructions on how to handle your child's behavior breakdowns as well as strategies for preventing them from happening in the first place (see section on positive reinforcement on page 160). He will also help you implement the food-chaining program at home as well as in a day care or school setting, if applicable.

Finally, the psychologist will work to make sure that your entire family agrees with all aspects of your child's food-chaining program and feels comfortable with the feeding team. If there are other stressors on the family, such as marital problems or unemployment, the psychologist is there to help you handle these issues.

WHAT'S YOUR CHILD'S LEARNING STYLE?

We all have a particular pattern of behavior that we use to learn new things. This pattern is called a learning style. While we don't approach every learning task exactly the same way, each of us develops a set of behaviors that we are most comfortable with. Below are the three most common learning styles. See if you recognize your child (or yourself) in one of these descriptions.

THE VISUAL LEARNER

Visual learners learn best by using their eyes to see information. They learn best by seeing words and numbers printed in text form, or by using graphics and pictures, observing real-life objects and events, and using maps, charts, graphs, and other visual aids. If your child is a visual learner, she will observe every little facial expression you make to figure out how you are responding to her. Your smiling eyes or mouth will be recognized as approval of what she's doing and encourage her to continue. A frown will make your child look away from you, perhaps with a head-down, pouty sort of look. By the same token, you can easily read her facial expressions to figure out how she is responding to what you are saying.

THE AUDITORY LEARNER

Auditory learners learn best by listening and talking. They take in information best through their sense of hearing. They learn reading and other subjects by listening to someone present information orally and by being allowed to discuss the topic and ask questions. Some auditory learners also learn best by involving music and sound effects. If your child is an auditory learner, she will be very sensitive to your voice tone and inflections. If your voice is too firm or you raise the pitch, she may sense that you are angry or frustrated with her. When you acknowledge her successes, she will know how sincere you are. If you correct her or tell her what to do repeatedly, she may think you are nagging and tune you out.

THE KINESTHETIC LEARNER

Kinesthetic learners learn best by moving their bodies, activating their large or small muscles as they learn. These are the "hands-on learners" or the "doers," who actually concentrate better and learn more easily when movement is involved. If your child is a kinesthetic learner, she will seem to have some part of her body moving constantly. She'll be a wiggler, a toucher, and want to be close to another person, whether that person wants it or not. She'll drum her fingers, rock, switch positions in a chair often, and likely be inattentive.

EVALUATING BEHAVIOR AT MEALS

When you are considering the behavior of your picky or problem eater, you should operate under the assumption that your child has a valid reason for protesting about food and look for evidence to support that. As we mentioned earlier in this chapter, we believe your child is behaving in negative ways because she's trying very hard to tell you something. The best way to start unraveling the mystery of your child's behavior is to be on the lookout for clues to why she is behaving negatively during mealtimes. Could she be unmotivated to eat because she drank a sippy cup full of milk or juice prior to the meal you are serving? Was she munching on crackers for the hour preceding the meal? You should also consider all of your child's activities leading up to mealtimes. What kind of day has she had? Has she been rushing around participating in after-school activities? Will she need to eat in the car as you take her to soccer practice or music class that evening?

Reading these clues can help you better understand your child's actions, and you can experiment with changes that may help her eat at mealtimes. For instance, if she had a sippy cup full of milk before dinner yesterday, don't give her one today and see if she seems more motivated to eat. Your observations will also give your child's feeding team unique insight into her behaviors at home, where she is most comfortable and unguarded. Not every mealtime is the right occasion to work on improving your child's feeding problem, and her feeding team needs to take her lifestyle and schedule into account and help you choose the best times to do so.

PROBLEMS THAT CAN TRIGGER FOOD REFUSALS

The following stories illustrate common feeding problems at different stages and how they can cause your child to begin refusing food. We'll show you how to recognize the negative behaviors that can help clue you in to what's going wrong and offer strategies to help you address them. On the surface, these stories seem to be about your child's readiness to master a particular skill or move on to a new stage of feeding. That is certainly part of the problem, but it can go far deeper. Your child's behavior may also be a response to an oral motor skill problem, which means your child will not outgrow them or just be "ready to eat" one day. It's important to speak quickly to her pediatrician about any problems you observe.

MILK SPILLS FROM YOUR BABY'S MOUTH DURING FEEDINGS

"Every time my baby takes her bottle, milk spills out the side of her mouth. I have to change her shirt after every feeding!" says Theresa of her three-month-old. It's not unusual for infants to be bottle-fed with a nipple that is too advanced for their abilities, which allows the liquid to flow into the baby's mouth too fast. This can be scary for babies because it makes them feel unsafe, as if they are drowning and can't get enough air. When the nipple flow is too fast and a baby feels she is in trouble, she will use a series of cues to indicate that something is wrong. She may clamp down on the nipple with her mouth, flattening it out to stop the flow of liquid. She may turn away from the bottle. She may push the nipple out of her mouth or allow liquid to spill from her mouth.

But if you don't know what to look for, it's not always easy to recognize that there is a problem. A caregiver may just think the

> **DID YOU KNOW?**
>
> Even though some pediatricians recommend doing so, it's dangerous to enlarge the hole of any nipple yourself. The cut could continue to enlarge over time and result in aspiration.

baby is being difficult. The fight between parent and baby over feeding will continue several times each day, and the baby learns with each feeding that she does not feel safe. She may start gagging as soon as she sees the bottle or it's placed in her mouth. In this example, the situation may be improved by switching to a slower-flowing nipple (see chapter 3 for advice on choosing the right nipple for your child).

DID YOU KNOW?

For infants born with a weak sucking reflex, many pediatricians recommend using a higher-flow nipple. However, it's important to know that the child's suck may strengthen in a few weeks or months, making the flow rate too rapid and therefore unsafe. It's very important to have your baby monitored by a speech or occupational therapist who specializes in feeding if she has problems feeding in the hospital.

YOUR BABY REFUSES TO BE SPOON-FED

"The day my baby turned four months old I offered her her first bite of baby food. She made a funny face and pushed the pureed apple right back out of her mouth. Now every time I try to spoon-feed her, she turns her face away," says Nancy. Sometimes older infants are transitioned from bottle- or breast-feeding to baby food before they have the skills to master this next level of feeding. Back in chapter 2, we described the tongue protrusion reflex and the role it can play in feeding disorders. This reflex is present in all babies until approximately six months of age, at which time you can introduce a spoon to the feeding process. But some pediatricians are telling parents to start spoon-feeding their babies as early as two to four months of age! This is completely inappropriate. The baby is being asked to do something that she does not possess the skills to do. A baby must have the ability to move the muscles of her cheeks, lips, and tongue in a coordinated manner to move the food to the back of her mouth for swallowing.

Some babies don't possess adequate head control to be spoon-fed yet, and others may be eating in high chairs that don't support their bodies well enough to enable them to eat with a spoon. The feeder may accidentally put the spoon too deep into the baby's mouth and gag her or scrape the spoon on the roof of her mouth. Or, she may force her to eat with the spoon. Imagine how awful that feels if you're not developmentally ready to spoon-feed yet. The baby may show that she is not ready by pushing the food out of her mouth, gagging, or turning away. The baby has a legitimate complaint—she doesn't feel safe.

If you see these cues and realize there is a problem, stop using the spoon and try again a few weeks down the road. When you try the spoon again, test your baby's readiness by resting the spoon on her lower lip and letting her suckle the spoon to move a small bite of food back into her mouth in a nonthreatening manner. If she still refuses the food and is older than six months of age, discuss this with your pediatrician.

DID YOU KNOW?

Spoons with a shallow bowl or a soft but firm bowl often work best for children who have sensory issues or gag easily.

YOUR BABY PUSHES HER SIPPY CUP AWAY

"Whenever I give my six-month-old a sippy cup, she cries, turns away, and fights the cup," says Ellen. These days many parents are told to introduce their babies to a cup as early as six months of age. This can be a surprising change for a baby—the nice, soft, manageable nipple that they can suck liquid out of is taken away and replaced with the hard spout of a cup. When the liquid comes out of the cup, it can overfill the baby's mouth, spill out of her mouth and back over the base of her tongue before she is ready to swallow. The baby's eyes water and she coughs. She may try to take another sip, but the same thing happens again. The baby learns that drinking from a cup causes her to choke on liquids, so she pushes it away with her hands or turns her head away when her parents offer it to her.

If your baby is pushing the cup away, there are several strategies you can try based on her specific behaviors. If you observe coughing spells or if your child does not sit well or have good head control, you may need to stop offering her the cup and try again a few weeks or even a month later. During this break, try giving your baby just the lid of the cup so she can mouth the spout and get used to the feel of it in her mouth. When you reintroduce the sippy cup, you may want to try a different product with a soft spout. Try putting just a small amount of liquid in the cup, thicken the liquid slightly with a little rice cereal (½ teaspoon per ounce), or add a little baby applesauce to apple juice so it won't flow so rapidly through the spout. Make sure your child is well positioned to drink. If she is in her high chair, make sure her body is properly supported and she's not slumping or leaning over in her chair. To improve her support, you can roll up some receiving blankets and put them on both sides of her body in the chair. This may help her use the muscles of her mouth more efficiently while drinking.

DID YOU KNOW?

You don't need to follow the "give your baby a sippy cup at six months" rule religiously. Only offer your baby a cup (preferably with a soft spout instead of a hard one) after she has demonstrated she has the skills for it—good head control and good bottle-feeding skills, which means no coughing or choking on bottle feeds.

YOUR BABY REFUSES TABLE FOODS

"My daughter eats baby food just fine, but when I offer her table foods, she gags and spits it out," says Bea of her 11-month-old. The transition to table foods is a major one for kids, and making the leap too soon can cause big problems. Eating seems like such an automatic and unconscious action to many of us, but in fact it's quite a complicated process. Table foods must be mashed up by our teeth and moved back to the center of the tongue before we are ready to swallow. Some children don't master this as quickly as others, or have medical problems that prevent them from mastering this (see chapter 3 for more information). Table foods don't break down in the mouth as easily as pureed foods, and pieces of food can stick to the back of a child's tongue and cause him to gag violently. Clearly this is a very unpleasant feeling. When this happens, Mom and Dad may panic and frighten their child with their reaction, which only compounds the problem. The child begins to feel that eating is dangerous for her and she doesn't like to do it.

Other cues that indicate your child is not ready to transition to table foods are if there is food left over in her mouth after she swallows; if food spills from her mouth while eating; if it takes multiple swallows for her to clear food from her throat; if she has congested or wet breathing while eating; or if she is "pill swallowing," which means she is attempting to swallow food whole without chewing.

Table foods also represent new textures that children must get used to. If your child has a sensory problem, she will tend to seek out food that has a uniform texture. Kids with sensory problems generally do not like food that changes as they chew it. For instance, some fruits and vegetables have a firm skin to bite through and a liquid texture underneath. These kids often do not like the aftertaste or aroma of vegetables. Meats are usually a challenge because kids with sensory problems find them difficult to swallow safely. Ten-year-old Chris told us that he "feels like he is swallowing a rock instead of food" when he tries to eat meat. Kids with sensory problems do not enjoy food that they can't count on being the same each time they eat it. They protest the only way they know how, by crying, refusing to eat, gagging, and even vomiting.

As these examples illustrate, many picky and problem eaters' negative behaviors may arise from sensory or medical issues that are interfering with your child's ability to eat, as opposed to a desire to misbehave.

DID YOU KNOW?

When transitioning your child from baby food to table foods, offer her meltable foods first, such as graham crackers or vanilla wafers with the ends dipped in pudding or baby food. These are often better options than Cheerios or bites of toast.

USING POSITIVE REINFORCEMENT AT THE TABLE

We strongly believe in the power of positive reinforcement to help improve kids' negative mealtime behaviors. Positive reinforcement not only builds self-esteem and inspires confidence in children, it's relatively easy to master. To use positive reinforcement, ignore your child's negative behaviors during meals (such as spitting food out, throwing food on the floor, and refusing to eat) and pay attention only to the behaviors that you want to support (such as taking bites of the food that you have offered or using utensils properly). This means not responding or reacting to your child's behavior in any way, not even to tell her to stop doing it. In fact, prodding your child to eat or offering her alternative foods is actually rewarding her for not eating. She knows that she has your attention and she calls the shots, which is what she wants.

Ignoring a bad behavior is the best way to extinguish it. Positive reinforcement teaches your child that she'll get no attention for her inappropriate or undesirable actions, but that you'll talk to her, clap for her, praise her, and generally engage with her when she behaves as you want her to. Usually it doesn't take long to see improvement in your child's behavior if you (and all caretakers) are consistent. A behavioral psychologist can help continually assess whether your positive reinforcement strategy is improving the situation.

When implementing positive reinforcement, it's important that you start by offering your child foods that you know she will eat. This way you can be sure that your child will understand how the process works—when she takes a bite of a food, she will get a positive reaction from you, and when she refuses to eat or misbehaves, she will get no reaction from you. If you try to begin with a food your child has never eaten before and she refuses to eat it, you will not have the opportunity to reward her positive behavior.

Here are some examples of negative behaviors and how positive reinforcement can be used to improve your child's behavior at mealtimes:

THROWING AND/OR SPITTING OUT FOOD

Eleven-month-old John loved to throw food from his high chair tray. Usually his mother, Patty, would pick up the food off the ground until she got so frustrated that she'd yell at John, and then take the food away from him. But this time, Patty doesn't tell him to stop throwing food—instead she offers John a small amount of food that she is confident he will eat. When he takes a bite of the food, his mother claps her hands and tells him how proud she is that he is eating like a big boy. John takes another bite of the food and his mother offers more verbal praise, telling him that he's doing a great job of eating. Then Patty gives him a piece of the food that he had originally thrown from his tray. When he eats it, she claps and praises him even more.

This is a perfect example of how positive reinforcement should work. Of course, sometimes things don't go so smoothly. For instance, let's say you offer your baby a small amount of a food that you are confident she will eat but she only takes a few bites and then begins throwing that food as well or spitting it out. Turn her high chair to face away from you for a minute. Do not talk to your child during this process. Then turn the high chair back to face you and offer your child the food again. If she eats it, praise her and continue the meal. If she throws or spits out the food again, turn the chair around and try once more. If your baby still throws or spits out food, you should remove all food from her tray, put an end to the meal, and try again next time.

This is hard for some parents to do because they feel guilty or anxious if their kids don't eat, but as you're scheduling your child's meals and snacks, your child won't go for very long without another opportunity to eat. And next time, she's more likely to accept the food.

Again, don't forget to look for clues as to why your baby may be behaving this way. If she's throwing or spitting out food after she's eaten an appropriate amount (see appendix 2, Feeding Your Baby and Young Child, for age-appropriate portion guidelines), then your baby may be signaling that she has eaten enough. You would then end your child's misbehavior by asking her to hand you pieces of food from her tray rather than throwing or spitting them out.

If your child is old enough to sit at the table, make sure she knows your mealtime expectations and what will occur if she doesn't meet them. Her meals should not last too long (no more than 15 minutes or so), and her body should be supported in her chair. You should also consider whether she is hungry or motivated to eat, the timing of meals (are you calling her to the table in the middle of a favorite TV show?), and whether she is drinking large amounts of liquids that may be dampening her appetite. All of these factors could cause your child to throw or spit out food. As with a baby, make sure you ignore attention-seeking behavior from your older child and praise good behavior.

DID YOU KNOW?

It may take an average of 10 exposures to a new food, paired with positive reinforcement, before a child will consistently accept the food.

CRYING DURING MEALS

Three-year-old Lily would cry at every meal that did not consist of her "favorite" foods. Her favorite foods are waffles, french fries, pizza, and chicken nuggets, so Lily was crying pretty often. Lily's mother, Ann, found this very frustrating, and she would often find herself shouting at Lily and in tears herself by the end of a meal. Ann decided to try using positive reinforcement to manage Lily's mealtime behavior. First she began offering one of Lily's favorite foods at every meal, so there was always something on her plate she was comfortable with. When Lily took a bite of food, Ann would praise Lily for eating successfully. For instance, when she took a bite of her chicken nugget, Ann would say, "You are eating like a big girl," or "Wow, you're doing a great job eating." When she cried or refused to try a food, Ann ignored her. When Lily's brother Simon ate something that Lily typically refused, such as peas, Ann would lavish him with praise. This actually encouraged Lily to try a taste of peas in order to earn Ann's attention. Lily's crying at the table diminished drastically when she realized how good it felt to please her mother.

If your child is crying at the table, and praising her for eating well is not working, continue eating your meal and ignore her. We know that this is difficult, but if you ask her to stop, you are positively reinforcing her negative behavior. If your child begins to calm down, you could say, "Good job settling down." You want your child to get the message that only acting appropriately will earn your attention.

Some kids become very distressed if they get messy during a

meal. If this is the case with your child, try putting a wet and a dry washcloth by his plate so he can wipe hands whenever he wants.

REFUSING TO SIT AT THE TABLE/ LEAVING THE TABLE DURING MEALS

Twelve-year-old Jesse won't sit at the dinner table longer than three minutes for a meal. It doesn't matter if his mother, Ginny, has cooked his favorite foods or something he refuses to eat—nothing will keep Jesse in his seat. He dances around the kitchen, then runs into the living room and back again, all the while grabbing bites of food off his plate. Ginny never knows when he's finished with his meals or how much he really eats. His behavior is distracting and annoying to the entire family.

If your child won't sit at the table for meals, it may be that the foods on the table are too visually challenging or there are too many aromas for him to handle. It also may be that he needs the sensory input he receives from standing and/or walking around the room to handle the mealtime experience. Try clearly stating your expectations of your child during mealtimes and devise a monitoring system before calling him to the table. For example, say to your child, "Your father and I are going to eat our pasta. When we are done, you may get up from the table. If you sit in your chair until we're finished, then we can watch a DVD after we clean up from dinner." Then, while your child is sitting at the table, offer him verbal praise, such as, "Thank you for sitting in your chair. We think you're doing a great job waiting for us to finish our pasta," or "I'm very proud of the way that you are sitting in your chair." After this is successful, slowly begin increasing the amount of time so he is sitting for longer periods.

Some children "act out" or try to leave the table because they don't feel secure or stable enough in their chair. They feel like they are sitting on a teeter-totter instead of a chair and this can be scary. Make sure that your child is seated properly with good body support during meals.

DISRUPTING OTHERS AT MEALTIME

Tom and Vivian find it very difficult to eat a meal with their five-year-old daughter, Kerry. It seems like all their focus must be on her at all times. If they try to have a conversation with each other or with Kerry's three-year-old brother, Josh, Kerry screeches, throws utensils, jumps up from the table and runs around the kitchen, or simply chants "Mommy" or "Daddy" until they turn their attention back to her. Mealtimes have become a circus. Disciplining Kerry hasn't worked, and Tom and Vivian are at the end of their rope.

If your child is disruptive at mealtime, it may be that he is using this strategy as a way to avoid eating and focusing on the food in front of him. He may also simply want everyone's attention on him at all times, like Kerry in the example above. In this type of situation, try ignoring your child, regardless of what he does to get your attention. Often when a child realizes that he can no longer turn the spotlight his way with bad behavior, he settles down. Keep in mind that it may take several meals before you see an improvement in your child's disruptive behavior.

If your child is very sensitive or has special needs, he may be acting disruptively because he can't stand the sound of other people chewing and eating. In fact, some kids with autism will put their hand over your mouth to dampen the sounds of your chewing. These children cannot tolerate the sounds others make around them while eating. Think about ways to seat your child away from a "noisy eater" or "lip smacker." Soft instrumental music at meals may also be helpful.

CAN'T FOCUS ON MEALS

Eighteen-month-old Jack needs to be distracted in order to eat during mealtimes. His mother doesn't try to force Jack to focus on eating—instead, she blows bubbles with each bite of food he takes. Sometimes she turns music on when Jack takes bites of food and turns it off if he begins to exhibit undesirable behaviors.

If you have a two- or three-year-old child with this type of feeding issue, you can create a "special" box of toys that your child can play with only if she complies with your mealtime rules, eats a desired portion of food, or tries a bite of a new food. You can make any rule you like as long as you clearly state your mealtime expectations to your child before the meal begins.

TIPS FOR IMPROVING YOUR OLDER CHILD'S AND TEENAGER'S MEALTIME BEHAVIOR

Reward your child with games. If you have an older child between the ages of four and seven or so, you could have her pick out a game or activity that she wishes to play after a successful meal. You can also create a sticker chart where, for example, 10 stickers wins her a toy or activity of her choice. Post the chart somewhere prominent so that after a successful meal, your child can place a sticker on it and feel proud. Sticker charts are great because they give children something motivating and rewarding to work toward.

Make your child part of mealtime routines. Your picky or problem eater should be part of your family's mealtime routines, such as washing hands, setting the table, serving food, and cleaning up. He should get no special dispensation for being a picky or problem eater.

Create and sign a contract. If your picky or problem eater is a preteen or teenager, create a contract that clearly states your expectations at mealtime, the rewards your child will receive for compliance, and consequences for his nonparticipation, which you both will sign. Make sure you are very specific, especially with regard to the food—for instance, when you set a goal together to eat a particular food, you should specify the portion size (¼ of a sandwich, 2 tablespoons of carrots, etc.) for the first try, the second try, and so forth. Make sure the contract states (and your child knows) that you are not going to verbally prompt him to eat throughout the meal.

As you've probably already surmised, positive reinforcement works by motivating and rewarding your child for behaving well. The key to success is to make sure that the reward you are offering is enough of a motivator for your child. In order to ensure this is the case, make your child part of deciding what the rewards will be. For instance, if you plan on using the "special" box of toys idea we mentioned earlier, take your child shopping with you at a dollar store or somewhere comparable for the items that will go into the "special" box.

Positive reinforcement can be a very effective tool for parents dealing with picky and problem eaters, but it will not necessarily solve every child's behavioral issues. Some children require a greater degree of behavioral intervention, and in cases such as these, only a behavioral psychologist is equipped to address their needs within a therapy setting.

FIVE TIPS FOR STAYING POSITIVE

Any type of disciplinary action, including positive reinforcement, can be difficult and emotional for parents. No one likes to be the bad guy, but now is the time to establish once and for all that you and your partner are in control, not your child. Sometimes it seems far easier to give in to your child to avoid a fight, but this will only lay the groundwork for far bigger and more devastating battles in the future. Being a parent is tough, so try using the following tips to help you stay strong and positive:

1. **Be consistent.** Consistently respond the same way every time you observe your child behaving in an unacceptable manner. If you give in to your child even once, you are telling her that if she continues to behave badly, you will eventually let her have her way.

2. **Look your child in the eye.** When speaking with your child, get down to her eye level—kneel if you have to. This will ensure that you have your child's full attention when you're talking to her.
3. **Say it only once.** Teach your child that you will say something *one time* and she must learn to listen. You don't want your child to ignore you until you raise your voice. Get down to your child's level, eye to eye, and tell her that from now on you will give her directions one time and she needs to learn to listen to you. The next time you tell the child something important, say her name to get her attention and make sure your directions are clear and short and the language you use is appropriate for your child's age and developmental level. Try holding up one finger as a cue to the idea of telling her something one time. If she doesn't listen, follow through and impose an immediate consequence, such as the loss of a toy or privilege. Never make a "If you don't do this, I will ___" statement that you don't intend to carry out. You must be extremely consistent, or the program won't work. It's probably hard to tell by the way she's acting, but your child wants you to assert your authority. Children need boundaries and limits to feel safe.
4. **Be clear about your expectations.** When you're cxplaining to your child what kind of behavior you expect from him, be as specific as possible. For

instance, when you go to the grocery store, don't just tell your child to "be good." That does not define what you expect. Instead, say "I want you to stay beside me while we're in the store." This way your child will know exactly what you want from him.

5. **Remember the golden rule of positive reinforcement.** Always ignore the behaviors that you want to go away and praise the behaviors that you want to see again.

HAVING FUN WITH FOOD

A big part of improving your child's behavior at mealtimes is finding ways to put the fun back into food. Most picky and problems eaters do not view mealtimes as fun, social events, which is what they should be. A more relaxed and fun approach to food and mealtimes will help your child begin to look forward to eating. This in turn will make her more receptive to trying new foods and help the food-chaining program succeed. Here are some ways you can help your child learn about food in an entertaining, nonthreatening manner:

LET'S GO SHOPPING

Anxiety can diminish a child's appetite. If you have difficulty getting your child to the table for a snack or a meal, or if she's anxious about the food you're giving her, introducing a fun, food-related activity before offering food can help her feel more comfortable. Cut pictures of food out of magazines or off the actual food packages and give them to your child to create a shopping list. Then, with your kitchen masquerading as a grocery store, make a game out of shopping for the foods on her list. We encourage you to be as silly as you want, perhaps hiding the carrots in your pots and pans cabinet and the peanut butter in the oven. (Note: You might want to hide your child's favorite snacks when playing this game—you don't want her to stumble upon the Goldfish crackers and then have to argue with her over eating some. This is supposed to be a calming activity, not an anxiety-provoking one!)

WHAT'S ON THE MENU?

Allowing your child some control over her food choices can help make mealtimes more pleasant. Make your child index cards with the names and pictures of different food choices. You can allow her to decide on one food for the meal or the entire meal. For instance, if you want your child to choose a fruit, give her one card with an apple on it and another card with a banana on it. We suggest you allow your child to choose between only two or three foods at the most. Giving her too many choices can be confusing.

You can also use the index cards to allow your child to tell you what food she wants to eat first, second, or third. However, if you're going to try this strategy, you may need to help your child make wise choices. For instance, if one of the foods you're serving is warm and should be eaten that way, don't allow your child to choose to eat it last, when it's cold. The taste of the food can change as it grows cold. You should also not allow your child to designate a new food to be eaten at the end of a meal. You don't want his anxiety about trying the new food to build as the meal progresses to the point where he won't touch it.

IT'S IN THE BAG

Many children with sensory processing problems (see chapter 4 for more information) gag when food touches their hands. If your child won't eat certain foods because touching them is unpleasant for her, helping her to explore foods by touching them is the first step toward overcoming the problem. Place plastic baggies over your child's hands and show her how she can manipulate and explore the food without getting her hands messy. Have her assist you in scooping or squeezing food items such as Easy Cheese, whipped cream, icing, pudding, Jell-O, cream cheese, or marshmallow cream in a plastic bag. Smell the food once it is in the baggie and encourage your child to do the same. Then seal the bag and suggest your child draw designs in the food through the baggie with her finger, or make tracks in the food by driving a toy car or train over the baggie. During these activities, discuss with your child how the food feels, sounds, and tastes.

You can also place dry food items such as cookies, crackers, or dry cereal in a baggie and discuss how the food changes as your child manipulates it. Suggest your child use a rolling pin to crush the dry food item, or a mallet to pulverize it into a powder. These strategies can also be used with mixed textured foods, such as Jell-O with fruit, cheesecake, or a casserole. Remember to talk with your child about what she is touching and how it would feel in her mouth. For instance, if you're talking about cheesecake, you could say, "When I take a bite of this cheesecake, it's very soft until my teeth hit the crust. Then it gets a little crunchy."

CHANGE THE SHAPE

Dig out those cookie cutters and show your child how fun it can be to change the shape of food. A cooked lasagna noodle, Jell-O, cheese, bread, lunch meat, pancakes, or a soft tortilla can all be cut into fun shapes. Engaging with food in this way helps your child become familiar with it through smell and touch. With close supervision, you can also allow your child to cut soft foods with a knife.

FUNKY PRESENTATION

Ditch those utensils and break out the fancy toothpicks—you know, the ones with the colorful frilly tops! Help your child arrange the food you've prepared for a snack into a fun design or shape—a circle of cheese and Cheetos makes a great sun. Grapes for eyes, a raisin for a nose, and strips of string cheese for a mouth and hair make a funny face! Buy some fun place mats and allow your child to determine which family member gets which place mat. Divided trays (the ones you used to see in the school lunchroom) or divided plates allow foods to be placed separately so that they don't touch one another and prevent the juice from a fruit or vegetable from mixing with other food items. Let your child decide which food item should go in which compartment.

LITTLE CHEFS

Let your child pour, stir, and scoop food into different containers or into the cooking apparatus as you're making a meal. We strongly encourage you to cook with your child to help her learn how different foods can be combined to make a new food, and how the smell of food changes as it cooks. Children who cook with their parents are proud of their participation and are often more apt to try a food that they have helped make. Plus, the more they know about how food is cooked, the less fearful they will be of food.

There are so many ways to incorporate fun learning activities about food into your day. These activities will help lighten the stress at meals for your entire family.

Bad mealtime behaviors can be among the toughest behaviors to handle. They cause huge amounts of stress and tension in families and can make the underlying feeding problems even harder to tackle. The advice and strategies in this chapter should go a long way toward helping you get your child's behavior both at the table and away from the table under control. Again, we encourage you to consult with a behavioral psychologist should these behaviors persist or worsen. In the next chapter, you will learn how to put the food-chaining solution into action.

CHAPTER 6

How Do I Get My Child to Try New Foods?

The Food-Chaining Solution

As an infant, Shawn ate very well—he took his bottle well and did fine with stage I and stage II baby foods. When he turned one, his mother, Natalie, started offering table foods. Shawn did not seem to like the texture of table foods. One day, he gagged and choked violently, and when Natalie tried to clear his mouth, vomited up his entire meal. Shawn was shaking and very distressed. He cried for a long time and had a hard time calming down after this frightening episode. The next day, when Natalie tried to place him in his high chair, Shawn did not want to eat. He clung to her neck and tried to climb back out of the chair. This marked the beginning of a long and difficult journey into Shawn's second year of life. Shawn learned to eat, but his diet consisted mainly of what

Natalie considered junk food. Shawn was easygoing and good-natured all the time— except at meals. There he seemed to be very distressed and he could not eat anything except his few "Shawn foods." The struggle continued as he reached his third birthday, except now there were concerns about his weight, and he still had not fully transitioned from baby food. Shawn ate about five foods well and preferred drinking his juice or milk over eating. Natalie tried everything, from coaxing Shawn to eat to forcing him, with no positive result. One night she and her husband decided to push it, and Shawn sat at the dinner table for two hours facing one bite of meat. They offered to buy him any toy in the toy store that very night if he would just take one bite. With tears running down his face, Shawn would bring the food up to his mouth, but he simply could not make himself take a bite. Everything fell apart that night during prayers, when Shawn told Natalie that he could not wait to be an angel, because angels do not have to eat food. Natalie called the pediatrician the next day and, after he evaluated Shawn, he referred him to a feeding team for help overcoming his issues with eating. It turned out that Shawn had a sensory processing disorder with a great deal of anxiety at mealtimes, and through a multidisciplinary therapy program and food chaining, he was able to eat and enjoy a much broader range of foods.

AT LAST WE arrive at the sixth and final step—creating food chains for your child. Now that any underlying medical, nutritional, sensory, behavioral, or oral motor issues your child has have been addressed, new foods can successfully be introduced into his diet. This chapter will help you determine what new foods to offer your child first and the best way to approach meals. Get ready to start expanding your child's diet!

WHAT IS A FOOD CHAIN?

As you know by now, there are very specific reasons why your child will only eat certain foods, but there is a way to help him accept a wider variety of foods. A food chain is a list of foods that have the same features (such as flavor, texture, or after-taste) as the ones he currently eats. Creating a food chain especially suited to your child's needs is a highly effective way to get him to accept new foods in a gradual and nonthreatening way. New foods are added to updated chains based on your child's reactions to previous new foods, and your child's diet plan is continually customized throughout his treatment.

HOW DOES FOOD CHAINING WORK?

Chaining is actually a pretty simple process. It's based on the idea that your child will eat what he likes. This is true of everyone; we all eat what we like. A food chain just introduces more foods that have the same flavors or features as foods that your child prefers.

First, you must look at the foods your child consistently eats at home, school, and/or day care, also known as his core diet, for patterns in taste, texture, temperature, and consistency. These foods all have something in common—perhaps they are all sweet, or hot, or bland, or crunchy, or salty.

You will also need to look at the foods your child used to eat and now rejects and has always rejected for patterns in order to understand what it is about these foods that your child doesn't like. (Your feeding team may try to offer foods your child used to eat again, to see if he will accept them, or modify previously eaten foods to see if he'll eat those instead. For instance, if your child used to accept pancakes, he might now accept waffles or French toast sticks instead.) You should examine these foods for patterns in texture, flavor, consistency, and temperature, the same way you would the foods your child currently accepts.

Once you and the feeding team have determined why your child accepts certain foods, the team will create food chains to help you broaden his diet (see page 199 in this chapter for sample food chain ideas and appendix 1 for sample food chains). You'll begin by introducing new foods that your child is very likely to eat because they are so similar to the ones he already likes. Once your child has expanded the foods he will eat in this way, you will move to the next level of the food chain, where you will begin to introduce new foods that are still similar to the ones your child likes, but have slightly different flavors and textures. Then you might add sauces, condiments, or dips to the chain.

Say, for instance, that your child loves to eat McDonald's chicken nuggets and your goal is to get him to eat grilled chicken. Your child's food chain would begin with your offering him different brands of chicken nuggets. It's a subtle change, but you are helping your child accept a greater variety of nuggets, which is the first step toward expanding his diet.

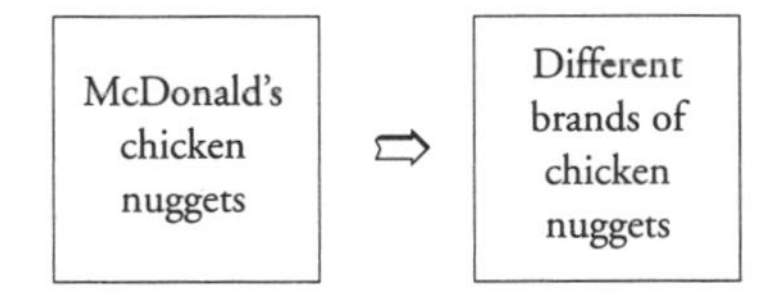

After he has accepted a few different brands of nuggets, then you would introduce chicken nuggets with slightly different tastes and textures. So if your child has only eaten lightly breaded nuggets, have him try some crunchy, more heavily battered nuggets. If he's only eaten plain nuggets up to this point, offer him nuggets with cheese blended into the breading. You could also offer your child chicken strips, to help him learn that the same foods can look different or be in different shapes. If he's hesitant to eat the chicken strips, you can cut them into pieces.

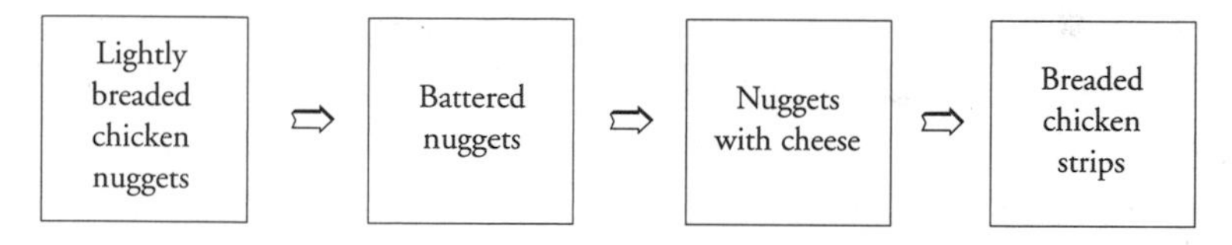

At this stage you would also offer your child other breaded items, such as popcorn shrimp, fried scallops, fish patties, or breaded pork tenderloin. Since you know he likes breaded chicken, it stands to reason that he might be successful eating other breaded meats. You're continuing to work on expanding chicken, but you're adding other types of food to his diet as well.

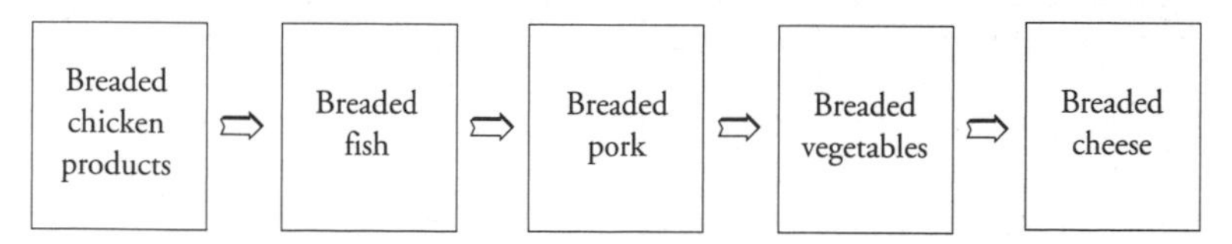

Then your child's food chain may call for sauces, condiments, or dips to be added to his food. (Some children cannot tolerate the mixed texture of a dip or condiments as dips, so they would only be on your child's food chain if he is likely to tolerate them. They are helpful but not crucial to food chaining.) Perhaps you would offer your child ketchup or barbecue sauce to dip his nuggets in. Then you would offer him a piece of grilled meat with an accepted sauce or condiment on it. The chain is complete—now your child is not only eating grilled chicken, but pork and seafood as well.

Chicken nugget with ketchup/ barbecue sauce
Grilled chicken with ketchup/ barbecue sauce
Grilled fish with ketchup/ barbecue sauce

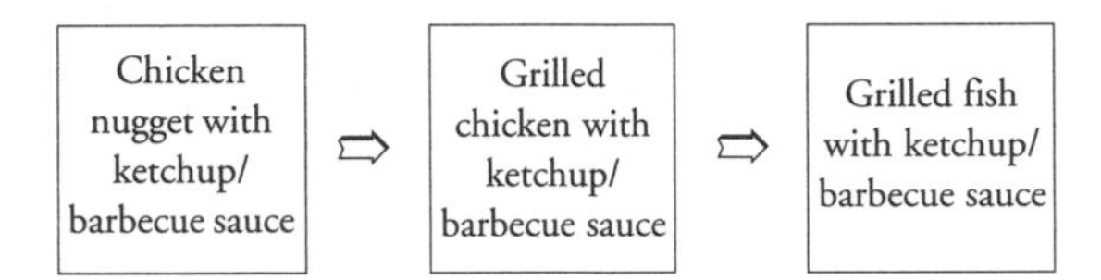

Or, if you think this might work better for your child, you might leave the chicken nuggets alone and try different sauces instead:

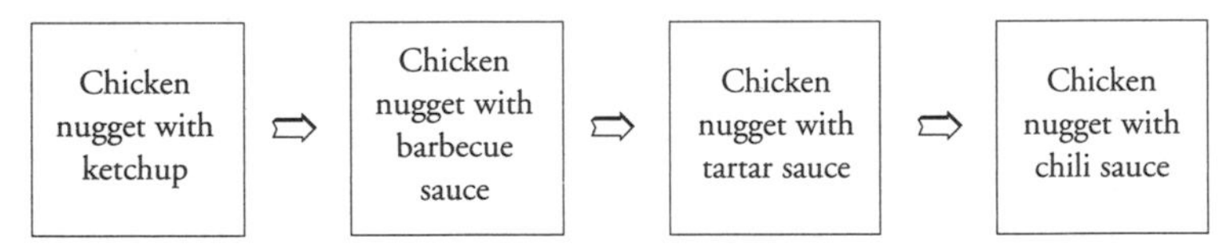

This is an example of a single food chain for one food. A food chain like the one above will be created for every food in your child's core diet. Usually only two or three foods are targeted at first, and a slightly modified version of those foods is offered one time a day.

It's important to understand that a food chain is not linear. It branches off in many different directions as your child accepts or rejects new foods and grows more tolerant of new tastes and textures. The following diagram, which begins with McDonald's french fries, helps illustrate the flexibility of a typical food chain:

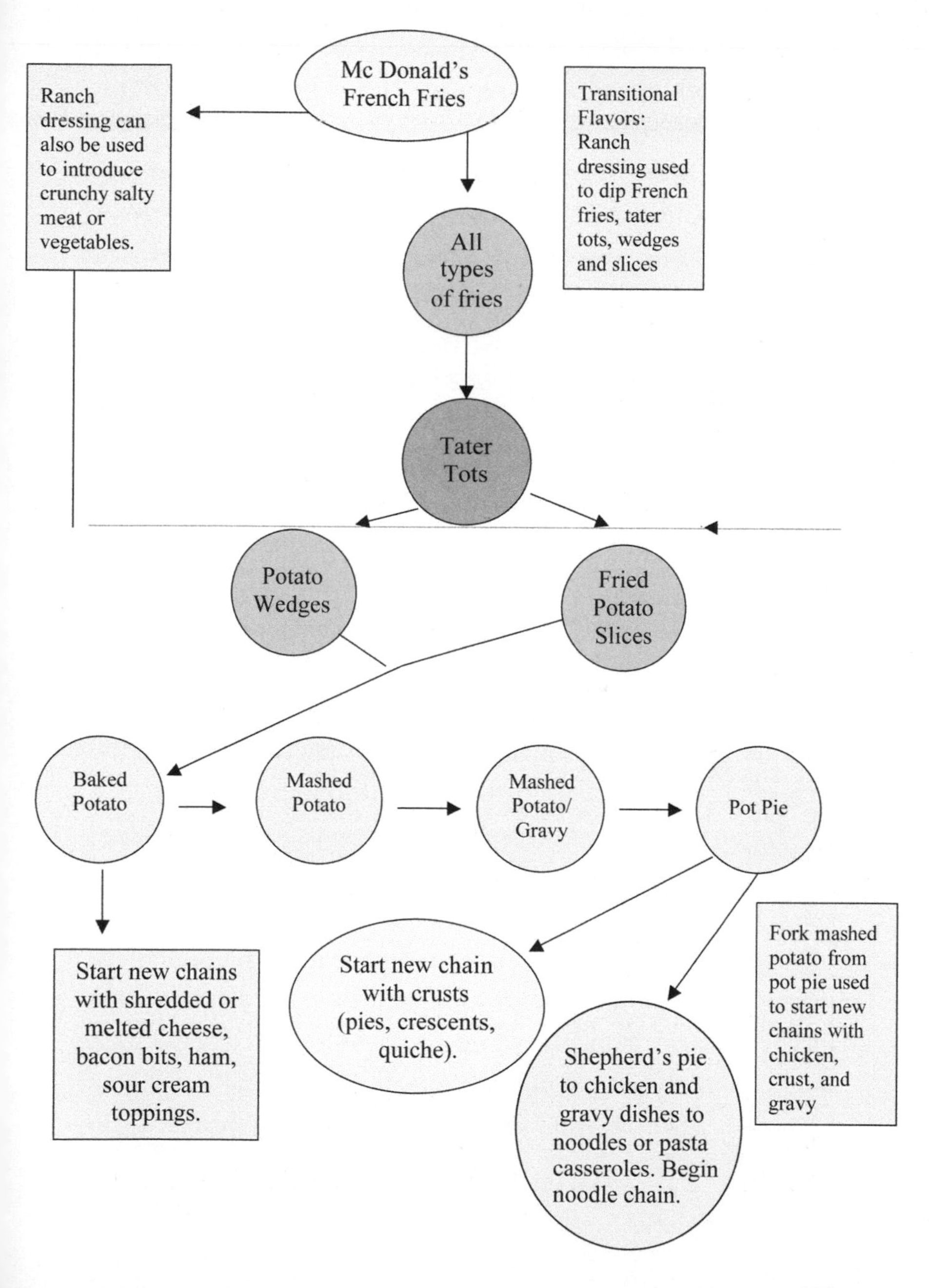
Mc Donald's French Fries
Ranch dressing can also be used to introduce crunchy salty meat or vegetables.
Transitional Flavors: Ranch dressing used to dip French fries, tater tots, wedges and slices
All types of fries
Tater Tots
Potato Wedges
Fried Potato Slices
Baked Potato
Mashed Potato
Mashed Potato/ Gravy
Pot Pie
Start new chains with shredded or melted cheese, bacon bits, ham, sour cream toppings.
Start new chain with crusts (pies, crescents, quiche).
Shepherd's pie to chicken and gravy dishes to noodles or pasta casseroles. Begin noodle chain.
Fork mashed potato from pot pie used to start new chains with chicken, crust, and gravy

You or your child should then rate every food on his chain with the food- chaining rating scale (see page 188 later in this chapter for more information) each time it is offered to him, which will dictate the pace and direction of his chain. Slowly but surely, you can continue to expand your child's food repertoire until he is consistently eating a healthy, balanced diet with a wider taste or texture preference.

Food chains are typically developed by the speech therapist, though they can also be developed by an occupational therapist or a dietitian who is trained to analyze the core diet and determine movements along the chains based on the rating scales. Food chains can be as structured or as unstructured as your child allows them to be. For instance, if your child shows interest in a food that someone is eating but that is not on their food chain, he should never be prevented from trying it. However, some kids and parents require strict structure and may want to use a food-chaining calendar. Plot new foods and serving amounts as well as core diet foods on a calendar to help you stay on track with the chain and continue rotating the foods that the child accepts.

Many parents have very specific goal foods for their children —usually meat, fruit, and vegetables, the hardest foods to tolerate. It's important to understand that food chaining is accomplished in small steps and it may take some time to achieve these goals. Food chaining is designed to expand your child's diet and provide him with more opportunities for a better diet. While your child may not be capable of reaching every goal you've set for him, food chaining will help him eat a wider variety of foods.

WHY IS FOOD CHAINING SO EFFECTIVE?

Food chaining is an effective treatment approach because it is based on your child's natural preferences and builds upon her successful eating experiences. Instead of trying to force your child to eat foods he does not find appealing or appetizing, you'll offer him foods similar to the ones he already likes. This significantly reduces the chances your child will reject the food or have an aversive response. The beauty of food chaining is that your child will be eating new foods, but it won't seem that way to him.

FOOD-CHAINING TERMINOLOGY

Here are the key terms a feeding team uses when talking about a child's food-chaining program. Use these definitions as a handy guide to help you better understand the process and keep up with the team's explanations of what's going on.

Core Diet: A core diet refers to foods your child eats reliably across all settings. These are the foods your child will accept no matter where he is—home, school, day care, a friend's house, and so forth.

Flavor Mapping: Flavor mapping refers to the team's analysis of your child's flavor preferences. The food-chaining intake form (see appendix 3) is used to evaluate each category of flavor that your child accepts. For example, if you categorized your child's foods and see that he accepts mostly salty foods and only one or two sweet foods, your child has a strong preference for salty flavors. This tells you and the feeding team that you should begin food chaining with spicy or other strong flavors before expanding sweet flavors. The team will also use your child's preferred flavors to help select new targeted foods. For example, if your child likes the flavor of cinnamon, the team may offer him cinnamon rolls, Taco Bell Cinnamon Twists, or cinnamon Pop-Tarts, or even introduce new foods such as a brown sugar–cinnamon or an apple-cinnamon pastry. Flavor mapping helps you know what flavors your child enjoys and helps expose him to a balance of different flavors as well as choose foods for your child's food chain that he is most likely to accept. Mapping is repeated over the course of treatment to monitor changes in your child's flavor preferences.

Flavor Masking: Flavor masking is the term used when a condiment or sauce is used to mask the taste of new foods for your child. Some picky and problem eaters like cheese sauce, ranch dressing, ketchup, or gravies, and they will accept bites of new foods if they are covered or dipped in a sauce or condiment. In cases like these, you might allow a sauce or condiment to be used at first to get the child to try the new food, but then decrease the amount of sauce over time. This allows the child to gradually experience more of the flavor of the targeted food and increases the chances he will accept it. Some children will not accept any dip or condiment, and you should not push your child if this is the case for him. He may surprise you and accept them later in treatment, but flavor masking works best with children who respond favorably to sauces and condiments.

Transitional Foods: Transitional foods are old favorites that are used to coax a child to try a new food. For instance, if your child likes corn muffins, you would offer him a bite of corn muffin in between bites of a new food. Transitional foods and drinks help to cleanse your child's palate and reduce the aftertaste effect that many picky and problem eaters find very aversive.

Surprise Foods: Surprise or "novel" foods are foods that are significantly different from your child's core diet. Surprise food may be offered once a week, and you should make your child aware that something special is coming. A surprise food can be a food you assemble, such as an ice cream sundae with all the different toppings, yogurt fruit smoothies, ice-based fruit drinks, or a chocolate fondue with small pieces of pound cake and fruits. It can be also be any type of fun food, such as pizza rolls, taquitos, chips and cheesy salsa dips. Ideally you should assemble or make the surprise food together so your child gains experience handling and making food. Be sure not to pressure your child to eat the surprise food. Many children will want to taste something they worked to cook. We try to make surprise foods a very fun and social eating experience, but we also use them to reduce a child's anxiety when presented with a new food. In therapy, the surprise food may be something we make together or it may be hidden from view in a special container. We have a large *Cat in the Hat*–style hat in our department and sometimes we hide the surprise food under the hat. We talk about the food item to see if the child can guess what it is, which gives us an opportunity to describe the features of the food.

Then the child, his parents, his siblings, and the therapist all eat the food together. (The child may only have to take a few bites.) We rate the food together using the food-chaining rating scale. We have had children find through surprise foods that they love kiwi or muffins or pecan pie. Surprise foods help your child get back to seeing food and eating as a fun, pleasurable activity.

THE FOOD-CHAINING RATING SCALE

Your child's feeding team will continually assess whether his food chain is working as it should with the food-chaining rating scale. This tool was developed by Cheri, Laura, and Sibyl to help feeding teams analyze a child's initial reactions to new foods and evaluate changes in a child's taste and texture preferences over time. The scale is a crucial part of food chaining because it helps you and your feeding team select new foods that your child is highly likely to accept as he moves forward, and the order in which these foods should be introduced. For instance, if your child begins giving cheese-flavored food items a favorable rating ("4" or above), the feeding team will likely incorporate cheese flavors into the new chains that they are writing for him. The ratings from the food-chaining scales directly impact the direction of future food chains.

Use the rating scale each time a new or modified food is introduced to your child and then every time it is offered from that point forward. For example, 11-year-old Eliot rated pizza a "4" the first time he tried it. When he tried it again two weeks later, he rated it a "7." The following week pizza was a "9," and then Eliot wanted it all the time.

Before you begin, you and your feeding team will set weekly

goals and determine mealtime rules, what foods will be introduced (you will typically expand three to five foods at a time), when they will be introduced, and the number of tastes your child is required to take. Each week you will share your child's food ratings with the team so they can determine which foods to modify next in the chain. As you'll see below, reactions to foods are rated on a scale of 1 to 10 (1 is low approval and 10 is high approval). Older children may also rate foods on a pediatric scale of 1 to 5. The pediatric scale is very child-friendly, and usually has pictures on it, such as a smiley face with hands thrown up for high approval and a face with a tongue sticking out for low approval.

The Food-Chaining Rating Scale

Strongly Dislikes									*Strongly Prefers*
1	2	3	4	5	6	7	8	9	10

1= Gags and/or vomits upon touching, smelling, or seeing the food
1+= Gags upon tasting the food
2= Chews the food or manipulates it briefly in the mouth
3= Chews the food, but strongly aversive to the taste, grimaces, refuses to try more
4= Chews and swallows the food, tolerates it, but doesn't enjoy it
5= Chews and swallows the food, tolerates it with a "so-so" reaction
6= Chews and swallows several bites of the food, no major grimace or reaction, but still hesitant
7= Chews and swallows several bites of the food with no hesitation, child appears relaxed
8= Chews and swallows the food, takes a small serving easily, pleasant look on the face
9= Chews and swallows the food, asks or reaches for more, appears to like the food very much
10= Chews and swallows the food, a strong favorite, accepts it at any time

We highly suggest that you keep a journal or a log of all your child's ratings so you can easily share it with the feeding team during your weekly check-ins.

BEFORE YOU GET STARTED

There are a few measures you should take before beginning your child's food chain.

Buy all the necessary products. If one or more of the specialists your child has seen suggested that you try a different type of spoon, cup, bottle, or nipple with your child, make sure you've bought the appropriate products and washed them so they are ready to be used. If you want to try using fun bowls, plates, or place mats with your child's favorite character on them to make mealtime more enticing, have them ready to go as well.

Stock your fridge. Sit down with your child's food chain and compare the list of foods, drinks, sauces, and condiments to what you've got in your refrigerator and pantry. For right now, focus on level I, in case the food chain is altered at some point down the line. If you're missing anything from the list, make a trip to the supermarket and stock up on what you need. Involve your child in the shopping so she can feel part of the process.

BEGINNING THE FOOD CHAIN

Once you've got everything ready to go and it's time to begin, take a deep breath and relax. It's very important that you start your child's food chain slowly. Don't try to rush things. We understand that this is easier said than done, but it's crucial

SOMETIMES A STEP FORWARD REQUIRES TAKING A STEP BACK

Once you've reached this step in the food-chaining process, you're probably very eager to get started and offer your child some actual new foods. But in some cases, a child is simply not ready to dive right in and expand his diet. You and the feeding team may first need to create a situation that's conducive to eating well. Sometimes that means taking a few weeks to help your child get used to a particular formula, bottle, or nipple that the team has recommended so he can establish foundational feeding skills. Other times that means taking the pressure off mealtimes by offering the foods your child already accepts at every meal and snack and not asking him to try any new foods at all for a few weeks. This will make mealtimes a lot less stressful and make your child more inclined to participate in meals and try new foods in the future. The point is that while you may feel like you're headed in the wrong direction, taking a step backward in this situation is not a bad thing. In fact, it is very beneficial. You are building a trusting feeding relationship between you and your child and establishing the idea that eating is a pleasant experience.

that you don't exert any pressure on your child to eat. The feeding team will give you very specific advice about the changes you should make to your child's diet, so all you need to do is follow them. Remember, feeding disorders take a long time to develop; therefore it will take time to undo the damage and for your child to learn new eating habits. It's also important that you take the time to make sure each positive change will last. Patience is the key to success. Working too fast or pushing your child too hard may very well do more harm than good.

Here are some important things to know about offering new foods:

1. **New foods are offered to picky and problem eaters based on what we call a "sensory hierarchy."** Your child must first be able to tolerate being in the same room as a new food. Then he must tolerate the sight of the new food, the aroma of the food, the feel of the food on his hands, and finally the taste by licking and then biting/chewing the food. Keep in mind that he may need to be exposed to a new food many times before he is ready to pick up the food and taste it or take a bite. (For this reason we recommend you don't cook enormous portions of new foods—most if it will probably go to waste.) This can be frustrating, but the good news is that each exposure to a new food teaches him about the food and helps him expand his sensory tolerance of food. Just keep telling yourself you are moving in the right direction.

2. **Never overwhelm your child by changing all his foods at once.** Your child needs to ease into each new small group of targeted foods or one or two foods individually. A good way to help him do this is to talk to him about a new food while you're cooking or serving

it to others, or, better yet, have him help you prepare or serve the food. Describe how the food feels, smells, and tastes.

3. **If a new food is not successful, consider whether you can modify it.** For example, if you're transitioning your baby to table food by adding small amounts of puree to baby food and your child rejects it, perhaps you added too much puree. You can reduce the amount of puree to as little as a ½ teaspoon if that's what your child can tolerate, and then increase the amount slowly over time. The important thing is not to stop trying when your child rejects a food. Often small changes to a food will make it acceptable to him.

DID YOU KNOW?

Adults can look at a food and predict how it will taste and feel in their mouths, but children cannot.

4. **Recognize that some foods are more challenging.** Meats such as roast, steak, beef, pork, and lunch meats or processed meats are particularly challenging for kids to eat because of their texture and consistency. Some children don't feel safe eating meat. Fruits and vegetables are also tough for many kids to eat because they

often have multiple textures and juices that spill out when bitten into. Your child's feeding team will likely target fruit, vegetables, and meats later in his food chain. You can still place a small, tablespoon-size portion of these foods on your child's plate or divided tray for exposure, but do not expect him to eat them at this point in his program.

TIPS FOR FOOD-CHAINING SUCCESS

Here are some general tips to help make food chaining as successful as possible for your child:

Give your child advance warnings. Don't just spring food on your child, even if you're following a routine schedule of meals and snacks. Give him some warning as to when mealtime or snack time will be. For example, if your child is watching TV, tell him that at the next commercial break you are going to turn off the TV and he will have a snack. Advance warnings of this kind tend to be better received by children than your walking over to the TV, turning it off in the middle of their show, and announcing snack time. Imagine how you would feel if someone turned off the TV in the middle of the season finale of your favorite show or the last minutes of the Super Bowl when the score is tied! Advance warnings not only show that you respect your child, they help you avoid getting into a major battle before the meal even begins.

Give your child choices. Giving your child a choice about what he eats will help him feel that he has some control over his feeding situation. For instance, if you are working with fruits, let your child choose between two fruits that you want him to eat.

Not every meal has to be part of the food chain. Not every meal is the best opportunity to work on your child's feeding goals. Pick a time when your child is not feeling tired or stressed, when you feel you have the best chance to gain his cooperation.

Time meals and snacks wisely. You've heard this before, but scheduling meals and snacks will be a huge help as you work to expand your child's diet. Meals and snacks must be spaced appropriately so that your child is hungry when you offer him food. Do not allow your child to snack or drink all day. This can dampen his appetite, and he may refuse to eat simply because he is not hungry at mealtime. If your child is not hungry, he will fight you through the entire meal.

Make the mealtime setting attractive to your child. We mention this above, but it bears repeating. Mealtime should be a fun and social event, so do your best to make it so for your child. For example, if he is a Thomas the Tank Engine fan, go pick out plates, place mats, utensils, and cups that feature Thomas. Make his food attractive by cutting it into different shapes with a cookie cutter or gussying it up with frilly toothpicks and little umbrellas.

FUN WITH PAINTING

When your child reaches the point in his food chain where he's experimenting with spreads, sauces, and condiments, here's a fun way to help him get used to them. Supply your child with a small paintbrush and allow him to paint a smiley face or other picture on an accepted food, such as a cracker. (Hint: Thicker spreads such as peanut butter or cheese can be thinned for easier spreading if you warm them slightly on the stove or in the microwave.)

If your child already accepts a condiment, sauce, or spread, pick a new food from his food chain and have him paint it with one of his choice. This way he will be using a transitional flavor to ease into accepting a new food.

Keep distractions to a minimum, unless directed otherwise. Don't distract your child in an effort to get him to eat unless you feel you really need to or his therapist counsels you to do so because of a sensory issue. Eliminate distractions and loud noise as best you can so your child can focus on eating. If you do need to use a distraction to get your child to eat, try blowing bubbles, playing music, giving verbal praise, or changing the presentation of the food. Don't offer tangible objects as distractions. You don't want to give your child a truck and then be forced to take it away from him when he refuses to eat because he wants to play.

Make a calendar of meals with your child. Allow your child to offer input on meals. For instance, each Sunday you could sit down with your child and create a calendar of meals for the upcoming week. Your child could help you decide what foods will make up the meals you prepare and on what days they should be eaten. A calendar will also help prepare your child for what is coming, much like the advance warnings we suggested above.

Make sure your child is comfortable at meals. Your child should be as comfortable as possible during mealtime. His clothing should be comfortable and his hair should be out of his face. You should have a wet and dry washcloth beside his plate to be used as needed. Make sure the chair supports your child under his feet and he is seated comfortably in an upright position (no slouching).

Motivate your child to succeed. If your have an older child or teenager, he needs to buy into the program and be motivated to change his eating behaviors in order to be successful. A good way to drive this concept home is to discuss why and how his feeding problem can negatively affect his social life, including dating, birthday parties, sleepovers, holidays, and big events such as homecoming or prom.

Rewards are also great motivators for kids. Consider making a deal with your child whereby he can earn special privileges at the end of each week of successful food chaining, such as renting a movie, going to the zoo, borrowing your car, and so forth. Or set up a point system where each successful meal earns him points toward purchasing a desired item or participating in an activity.

Shift the focus off your child at mealtime. Often the biggest challenge when food chaining with older children is reducing the amount of attention you give them for not eating. Picky and problem eaters are usually the center of attention at mealtimes because their parents are concerned about how much they are eating. Kids love being the center of attention, so losing that focus does not usually sit well with them. However, paying attention to your child for not eating will only perpetuate his feeding problems. You are in essence rewarding him for not eating. See chapter 5 for tips on using positive reinforcement during mealtimes.

Don't reward negative behavior. If your child chooses well and follows the program guidelines, by all means praise his behavior. If your child chooses poorly and does not meet your expectations at a meal, make sure he faces the consequences. If he's hungry before bedtime, offer him a less than desirable snack, such as a small amount of cereal or a granola bar or a piece of fruit. Don't give him the ice cream and cookies he's probably asking you for. If you do, your child will believe that he doesn't have to eat and he will still get a treat before bed. That will sabotage his food chain and his entire feeding program and he will never get better. Consequences will help your child make better choices in the future.

The whole family should support your child's program. This is especially true for older children and teenagers, because they must overcome a more established pattern of eating. All kids need the consistent support of their efforts to change from every family member.

SAMPLE FOOD CHAINS

ACCEPTED FOODS AND SUGGESTED MODIFICATIONS

Bacon

- Try other brands of bacon.
- You may use bacon grease to fry ham steak.
- Try foods that are similar in flavor to bacon such as ham, summer sausage, pepperoni, fried bologna, pastrami. Select one and offer a bite or two with your child's other regular foods and see if she shows interest at this time.

Beef jerky

Make sure it is safe for your child to swallow this food.

- Summer sausage cut thin is a good alternative to jerky.
- Also consider offering pepperoni or salami along with jerky.

Carnation Instant Breakfast

- Add Hershey's chocolate or strawberry syrup or cocoa mix for flavor change. Start small at ¼ to ½ tsp of syrup, or add ¼ cup ice cream, stir well, and increase amount as needed. This is an excellent source of nutrition until you can expand his diet further or introduce a caloric supplement such as PediaSure, Nutren Junior, or Kindercal.

Cheerios

Offer MultiGrain Cheerios, Honey Nut Cheerios, Yogurt Burst Cheerios, Froot Loops, or Trix cereal.

Cookies with sprinkles

Add sprinkles to other foods (homemade toppings, toast, doughnuts, pastries, pancakes).

French toast

Try a variety of different brands of French toast or offer it with powdered sugar or flavored syrup. You could also try cinnamon rolls, pancakes, or waffles.

Froot Loops

- Rotate Froot Loops with a few pieces of other cereal, such as Apple Jacks, Trix, or Kaboom.
- Try Kix, Rice Chex, or other crunchy cereals, and flavored Cheerios.
- If your child eats Froot Loops cereal bars, offer Rice Krispie treats.

Garlic bread

- Try different brands of garlic bread, garlic toast, or Texas toast.
- Garlic bread sticks, Pizza Hut or other restaurant-style bread sticks, hot rolls with garlic butter, garlic cheese bread.
- Try thick-crust pizzas, Stouffer's pizza bread, and pizza breads. Pizza is great because you can add many new foods to it.
- Hard seasoned bread sticks, croutons, seasoned crackers (garlic or other seasonings) may be offered to expose your child to a more challenging texture.

Homemade granola

Make homemade granola together and offer store-bought granola or cereal with granola added. Also try offering a granola bar.

Juice, V8 splash

- Try a variety of drinks with citrus taste.
- Offer a variety of juices to give the child a variety of taste stimulation.

Pepperoni pizza

- Pepperoni pizza can be modified by adding bacon, ham, or Canadian bacon to the pizza.
- Bacon pizzas with finely chopped bacon are likely to be accepted.
- Fine ground sausage may also be accepted.
- Zucchini and squash can be pureed and added to sauce (use his preferred toppings, too) for homemade pizza.
- Spaghetti sauce may be accepted since he shows a preference for pizza sauce.

Popcorn

Offer flavored popcorn or try something new, like adding a few drops of Tabasco sauce to popcorn. Try offering a popcorn ball or hull-less popcorn made from vegetables.

Potato chips

- Offer all brands of chips, shoestring potatoes, and Pringles (BBQ, etc). Next offer pretzels, cheese curls, Bugles, or Doritos.
- Offering vegetable chips, crackers, or Pirate's Booty (made from vegetables) is a good way to introduce vegetable flavors.

Tip: A great deal can be achieved by adding variety to a food that your child already accepts. We often use foods that are familiar, such as chips and seasoned crackers, to offer a variety of tastes and keep the child from getting too restricted in what he will accept.

Pretzel

Yogurt-dipped pretzels, chocolate-dipped pretzels or different pretzel shapes, such as pretzel sticks and twists. If your child accepts dips or condiments, try having her dip pretzels in cheese dip, cream cheese dip, mustard, caramel, peanut butter, or chocolate.

Yogurt

Offer yogurt smoothies with pureed fresh fruit or just a small amount of juice added. You can add into your drink first and then show him as you add new juices or flavors to his drink. If he is not ready, just alter your drink at first.

Puree a small amount of fruit and add to yogurts, or mix in to yogurt smoothies. Also try drinkable yogurts.

In order to give you the fullest possible picture of how food chains work for every age group, we've provided complete food-chaining programs for a toddler and a school-age child below, plus programs for an infant, a young child, and a teenager in appendix 1. These are real food-chaining programs, created for children who have been treated by our feeding team. The names have been changed to protect their privacy.

BRADEN'S FOOD-CHAINING PROGRAM

Two-year-old Braden was demonstrating behaviors at meals that concerned his family and pediatrician. He was rejecting more and more foods that he had previously accepted. He did not appear hungry at meals; he often did not wish to eat in the morning hours and wanted his cup instead. Braden's mother felt her control of meals was "slipping away" and she was feeling an increasing level of anxiety as she prepared meals. Since Braden refused to eat at mealtime, she followed him around the house with snacks, or food was brought to the living room in front of the television after a behavior breakdown at the table.

Braden's parents did not feel comfortable with this, but they felt he needed to eat. Sleep issues were also emerging, with Braden waking at night and wanting his cup. Braden always accepted his cup and liked to drink from it while he walked around the house.

Family Goal: Braden's family wants to improve Braden's nutrition, learn how to handle his mealtime behavior, and sit down at meals as a family.

Step 1: Medical Evaluation Braden suffers from significant gastroesophageal reflux, which began in infancy. His reflux appears to have contributed to his feeding aversion. Prior to coming to our clinic Braden was on Zantac; however, this medication was not strong enough and he was switched to Prevacid. Braden's reflux may be behind his refusal to eat in the morning hours, his preference for drinking, and his sleep issues.

Step 2: Nutrition Evaluation Braden eats a variety of foods, but he grazes during the day and doesn't have scheduled meals or snacks. His liquid intake is adequate but also not scheduled. His nutritional status and weight are fine, so we were able to allow him some space to develop his self-feeding skills and a feeling of independence when eating, which is a developmentally appropriate stage of feeding for him. The nutritionist discussed appropriate portion sizes for Braden (1 to 2 tablespoons of each food item, with two to three foods from different food groups offered at each meal). She recommended scheduling his meals, snacks, and liquids to help manipulate his appetite. Braden's mealtimes should be limited to 20 to 30 minutes and snacks to 10 to 15 minutes. Scheduled meals and snacks and gentle appetite manipulation should increase Braden's intake during the day and improve his sleep patterns. He may be waking up because he is hungry. A multivitamin is recommended if Braden will accept it.

Step 3: Feeding Evaluation Braden's oral motor skills are within normal limits. Braden's parents should encourage him to self-feed by offering finger foods and easy-to-spoonfeed items, as he needs to develop these skills. The speech therapist suggested using the double spooning technique; both Braden and the parent feeding him would get a spoon and have a chance to spoon food into his mouth (this is a short-term measure and should be used only when needed). This would help Braden feel in charge at meals while ensuring that he takes in an adequate amount of food. The therapist also advised Braden's parents to allow him to be independent at meals by letting him self-feed as much as possible. He needs to master this skill, and his behavior may be caused by his inability to achieve a state of independence at meals.

Step 4: Sensory Evaluation Braden has strong sensory preferences about foods. He accepts certain foods for a reason. He should be encouraged to inspect food visually, by smell, by touch, and finally by taste (licking or actually taking a bite). Braden's parents should try offering one new food paired with an accepted food at one snack time each day at first. They need to be careful not to overwhelm him with change, or he may shut down.

Step 5: Behavioral Evaluation Braden is a typically developing toddler. At the time of his evaluation, Braden was going through a stage where he fought his parents for control at meals. The psychologist found that Braden's parents were not consistent in their approach to his food refusals. His father gave in and let him eat what he wanted, and his mother pushed him to eat new foods but didn't follow through when he misbehaved at mealtimes. Bringing food into the living room in front of the television was a major red flag. Braden's negative behaviors at meals were being rewarded when he was allowed to leave the table, graze, and watch TV. He also had his parents' full attention at every meal. He was increasingly in control of each mealtime.

The psychologist found that Braden accepted a wider variety of foods when he was at day care. But when his parents attempted to offer him the foods he accepted at day care, Braden wouldn't eat them. The behavioral evaluation made clear that a consistent routine for meals, eating with other children, and self-feeding opportunities are important to the success of Braden's meals. The psychologist advised Braden's parents to approach meals without anxiety and to allow natural consequences to occur if Braden refused to eat (meaning he'd have to wait until the next scheduled snack or meal to eat again). She also encouraged Braden's parents to praise positive eating behaviors (see chapter 5 for more information on positive reinforcement during mealtimes) and model good eating behaviors. Braden might show interest in new foods if he saw others enjoy them.

Step 6: The Food Chains Braden shows a strong preference for peanut butter and crunchy foods, but foods are dropping out of his food repertoire quickly. Our goal is to prevent any further loss of foods and improve nutrition. Braden accepted a good variety of foods at one time, so we are optimistic that he will do so again. We encouraged Braden's parents to start slow, with a no-pressure approach.

BRADEN'S CORE DIET

Texture preference: Crunchy foods and smooth peanut butter. Braden enjoys food that gives him sensory feedback in his mouth. Crunchy food is easily crushed by the teeth, and the texture does not change while chewing.

Taste preference: Salty foods.
Temperature preference: Warm or room-temperature foods.

Accepted breads: Ritz crackers, Club crackers, and Cheez-Its.
Modifications: Try a variety of crackers, Ritz Bits with peanut butter or cheese, cheddar cheese crackers, Goldfish crackers, and Cheetos. Offer Braden thin-crust pizza and whole-wheat toast cut into tiny pieces.

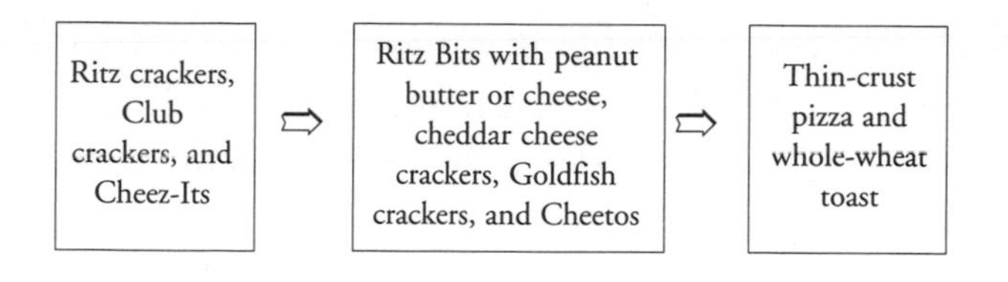

Accepted meats: Fried chicken, chicken nuggets, and fried fish.

Modifications: Do not try to modify meats excessively at this stage of treatment. Simply keep rotating the meats Braden accepts. You can try offering a variety of chicken nuggets and strips, fish sticks or patties, such as the ones sold at Long John Silver's or McDonald's. Later we will try other breaded meats such as fried scallops, mild fish, and pork tenderloin.

New food idea: Offer bacon (baked on a cookie sheet at 400° F for about 10 to 12 minutes) because Braden likes crunchy, salty-type foods. If bacon is accepted you can also try thin fried ham, pepperoni, or salami.

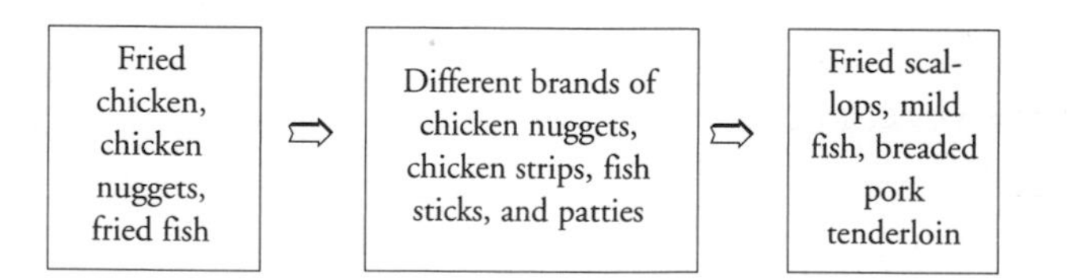

Accepted cereals/breakfast foods: Cheerios and Honey-Comb cereal. He has previously accepted waffles.

Modifications: Expand cereals from regular Cheerios and Honey-Comb to flavored Cheerios, Rice Chex, Rice Krispies, Kix, Froot Loops, and so forth as tolerated. Offer plain Pop-Tarts with strawberry or grape filling as these are fruit flavors Braden is likely to accept. Waffles can be offered with butter and/or jelly or cut into pieces to dip in maple syrup. You can also try blueberry or fruit-flavored syrup. Try offering French toast sticks and thin pancakes that are easy to eat. If you make thin pancakes, try pureeing a fruit, such as banana, blueberry, or strawberry, and adding it to the pancake batter. Start with one tablespoon at a time. This gives Braden fruit flavors in an accepted texture of food.

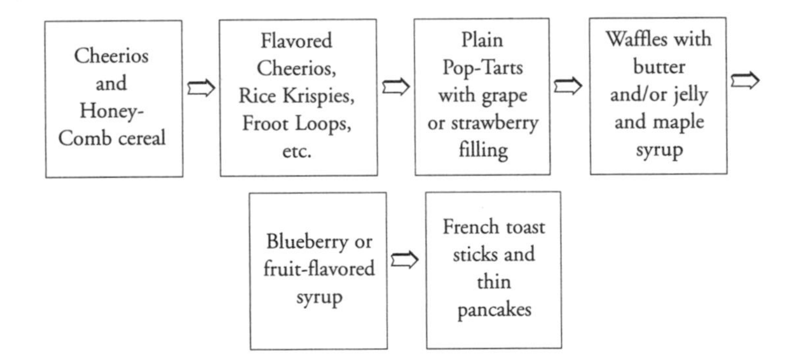

Accepted vegetables: Braden accepts green beans, sweet potatoes, potatoes, and carrots.
Modifications: Offer green bean casserole with Durkee onions over the top (crushed or whole) to give a salty, crunchy taste to an accepted vegetable. Try baking a sweet potato and adding maple syrup or brown sugar and butter. (You may want to add a crunchy brown sugar topping over whipped sweet potatoes, as well.) Sweet baby carrots can be cooked and offered cut into narrow strips. Since Braden accepts potatoes in

the form of french fries and mashed potatoes, he will very likely accept potatoes in other forms as well, such as tater tots, hash browns, fried potatoes, twice-baked potatoes, cheddar potatoes, and au gratin potatoes. This will add variety to his diet and improve his acceptance of novel foods, or foods very different from the ones in his current diet.

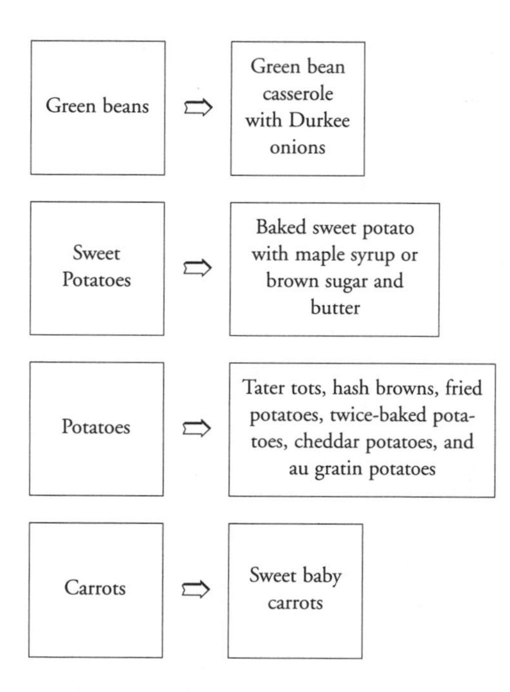

Accepted pasta: Kraft macaroni and cheese.
Modifications: Keep offering macaroni and cheese, but start using the Kraft powdered cheese mix on other types of pasta, such as elbow macaroni, bow ties, and spirals. Work toward getting Braden to accept more traditional macaroni and cheese

recipes. Try offering Braden hamburger meat. Cook the hamburger and then process the meat in the blender so it's very fine. (The consistency should be like the meat in Taco Bell tacos.) If Braden accepts meat this way, you can offer him any type of hamburger dish, such as chili, tacos, casseroles, and sloppy joes.

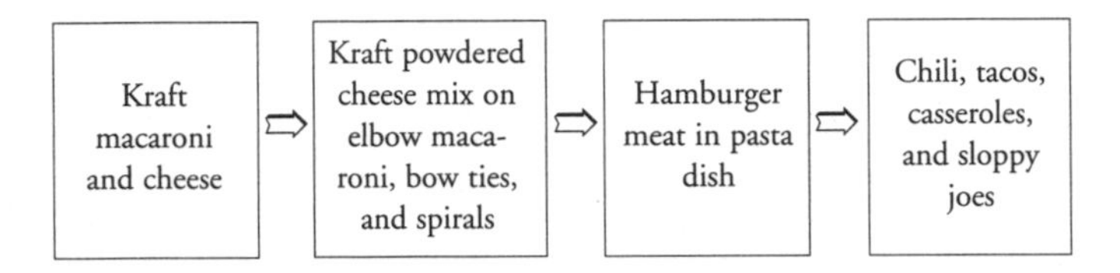

Accepted soups: Beef stew and chicken noodle soup
Modifications: Continue offering these soups, but also try chicken and dumplings or a spicy taco soup.

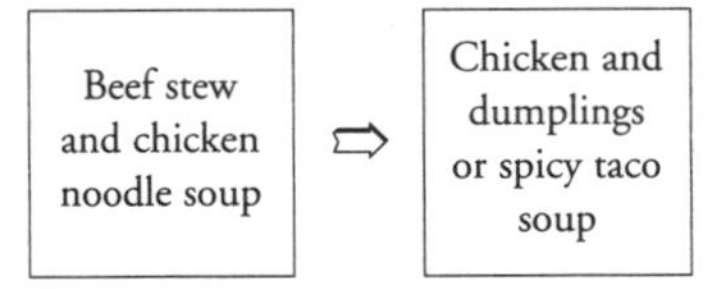

Accepted peanut butter: Smooth and creamy
Modifications: Offer peanut butter on a variety of foods, such as toast, crackers, breads, mini bagels, apple (thin slices), and banana (not too ripe). Braden may also accept a peanut butter smoothie or peanut butter cookies. As you progress, add new flavors to peanut butter, such as different jellies and jams.

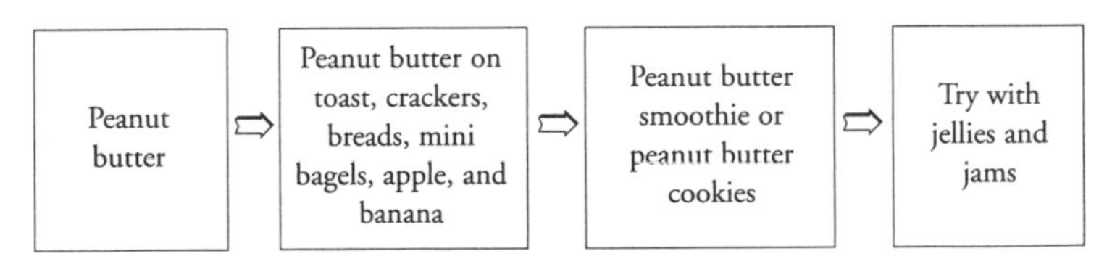

MELISSA'S FOOD-CHAINING PROGRAM

Eight-year-old Melissa's parents brought her to see us because she was eating a very limited number of foods. When they tried to get Melissa to eat new foods, she would gag or vomit. Note that Melissa's food-chaining program is set up differently than Braden's because of her age and the complexity of her problems.

Family Goal: Melissa's parents want her to learn how to accept more foods, particularly meat, fruit, and vegetables.

Step 1: Medical Evaluation Melissa is in good health. Her medical and developmental history is normal.

Step 2: Nutritional Evaluation Melissa eats six foods and drinks three liquids—water, juice, and occasionally milk. Her favorite foods are pasta with cheese and butter, chocolate pudding, chocolate milk, Cheez-Its, Goldfish, and corn bread. Many foods have dropped out of Melissa's food repertoire. Her least favorite foods are meats, vegetables, and fruits. Melissa prefers foods that have a uniform texture and maintain that texture during chewing. Melissa selects foods based on her ability to tolerate them from a sensory perspective. She exhibits strong patterns in her preferences.

Step 3: Feeding Evaluation Melissa's oral motor feeding skills are normal and her oral reflexes are intact.

Step 4: Sensory Evaluation Melissa appears to have very significant sensory issues that require assessment. However, her parents are focused on her behavioral feeding issues and have not yet consented to a sensory evaluation. At this point we suggest that Melissa participate in food preparation to help desensitize her to the sensory properties of food.

Step 5: Behavioral Assessment Melissa is a very bright girl. She is interested in health and appears to be very interested in the nutrition assessment and information provided to her family by the dietitian. Melissa does not appear to enjoy meals at all. She gags on food and often cries through meals. Her parents have tried many different behavioral techniques to help her broaden her food repertoire, but no approach was consistently implemented over time. They are frustrated because they feel nothing has worked and meals have become too stressful.

All of Melissa's siblings attended her behavioral assessment and complained about Melissa's eating patterns. Melissa was receiving positive and negative attention for her eating issues and she was the focus of her entire family during all meals. This may have been increasing the tension at meals and adding to Melissa's reluctance to eat. Melissa's family needs time to decompress and learn how to let meals simply be about eating.

At first, Melissa should be offered only food she is highly likely to tolerate at meals to maximize her chances of success. Her meals and snacks should be scheduled. The psychologist recommends that the entire family participate in therapy so she can explain to them Melissa's food issues and her sensory concerns and show them how to support her as she works to increase her food repertoire. The psychologist will monitor Melissa closely in direct treatment sessions with her family.

Step 6: The Food Chain Melissa prefers foods that are crunchy and chewy and that maintain a uniform texture during biting and chewing. Melissa prefers tastes that are salty and responds well to strongly flavored foods.

MELISSA'S CORE DIET

Accepted foods: Since Melissa accepts more foods than Braden in her core diet, we categorized her food preferences by food group.

> **Breads:** Crackers (Cheez-Its, Goldfish, and Doritos), corn bread, pizza without crust, frozen pancakes, waffles (peels away outer ring on waffle), bagels, cupcakes, Texas toast, garlic bread, biscuits, doughnuts, dry cereals, and Pop-Tarts.
>
> **Pasta/Rice:** Pasta without sauce (she adds butter and a small amount of Parmesan cheese), plain white rice, macaroni and cheese, occasionally pasta with Alfredo sauce or small amount of red sauce.
>
> **Meats:** Chicken strips, chicken nuggets, popcorn chicken (from McDonald's, Sonic, and Tyson).

Dairy: American, Parmesan, mozzarella cheeses, chocolate pudding.

Vegetables: No easily accepted vegetables. Melissa eats corn, she attempted broccoli once (one bite), and eats carrots occasionally.

Fruits: No easily accepted fruits, though she has tried an apple pastry. Therefore, apple flavor will be explored as this appears to be the fruit taste Melissa is most likely to accept.

Accepted liquids: Melissa will drink water, milk, and apple and grape juices. She prefers water and juice over milk. (Milk tends to coat the throat, which makes it less pleasurable for many kids to consume.) Her liquid intake is normal.

TEAM RECOMMENDATIONS

General

Meals should not be focused on Melissa. She is a very bright child and increased focus may encourage more negative behaviors at meals. Meals need to return to a social, enjoyable experience focused on the family that remains within the normal time range for a child Melissa's age.

Approach meals with the expectation that Melissa will eat. Provide her with food at regular intervals (see Meal Length below). If Melissa chooses not to eat, make sure she faces the consequences (hunger). To begin, we will offer her foods that her sensory system can tolerate and not challenge her with foods that she will find aversive. As we work with Melissa over time, we will expand her tolerance for foods outside of her core diet.

Meal Length

Meals should last approximately 20 to 25 minutes. Offer three meals per day. Two to three snacks can be offered and should last approximately 15 minutes. Try to have at least 2.5 to 3 hours between meals and snacks to gently stimulate appetite.

What to Offer at Meals

Foods Offer only foods in the core diet at first to allow a cooling-off period and normalize Melissa's meal experiences as much as possible. Rotate these foods to provide variety as much as possible. When you reach the point where mealtimes are without conflict and she is back to eating her core diet in an acceptable time frame of 20 to 30 minutes, offer her core diet items as well as foods in the level I modification lists (see the food-chaining modification chart below).

For example, at breakfast rotate dry cereals, Pop-Tarts, peanut butter on bagels, French toast, waffles, and pancakes. Then move into the modifications to these food items based on how she rates them on the rating scales.

At lunch and dinner, Melissa likes a wide variety of breads and crackers, and she will accept varying types of pasta (spaghetti, pasta with butter and cheese, macaroni and cheese). Many children do not like sauce on their pasta. It's fine to allow this to continue and not target pasta with sauce in treatment. Chicken nuggets, chicken strips, and popcorn chicken can be offered with a variety of pastas and breads. Rotating preferred foods prevents Melissa from developing a food jag, where she eats one food exclusively.

You can also offer a tablespoon of a fruit or a vegetable (corn or carrots, since she has previously accepted these), but do not push her to eat them at this time.

Liquids Offer Melissa milk with meals. She should only be offered water (two to four ounces) between meals to help manipulate her appetite and prevent her from filling up on liquids. Melissa may prefer juice with two tablespoons of orange sherbet instead of milk. Adding sherbet changes the consistency of the milk and prevents excessive coating in the throat. We will gradually work toward improving her tolerance of milk products.

Vitamins Try Scooby-Doo Fizzy Vites (picky and problem eaters tend to enjoy the sensory feedback these vitamins offer and they don't have a strong aftertaste).

Feeding Therapy
Weekly sessions with the feeding specialist are recommended to help Melissa start her treatment program and to further evaluate her feeding issues.

Occupational Therapy Referral
Sensory processing evaluation and treatment by an occupational therapist is strongly recommended.

Psychology Referral
Melissa and her family will meet with our team psychologist to

provide support to all family members, help with communication at meals, set reasonable rules and consequences, and assist with communication with Melissa's school regarding lunch and snack programs.

MELISSA'S FOOD CHAINS

Select one or two foods to modify initially. Do not rush through the program or change all foods at once. Progress from level I to level II foods as tolerated. It may take several months for Melissa to complete this food chain. Use the parent and child rating scales to measure Melissa's reactions to new foods. Once you reach level II, do not be afraid to offer novel or surprise foods.

Core Diet Items and Modifications

Meats

- Chicken nuggets
- Chicken strips
- Popcorn chicken

Level I

- Offer a variety of brands and types of chicken nuggets/strips/popcorn chicken and chicken patties. Schwan's or Tyson's can be offered at home or you can bread and cook your own.
- After Melissa accepts more variety, offer a chicken leg as an alternative.

Level II

- Offer a variety of flavors and textures of chicken nuggets and strips. Sonic, KFC, Hardee's, McDonald's, Long John Silver's, Arby's, Popeyes, , and other restaurants offer a variety of chicken products that she may accept. You can also try any grocery-store brand.

- Offer breaded seafood (popcorn shrimp or scallops, fish patty from McDonald's, etc.)
- If she will accept a dip or condiment, this may help us transition her eventually to baked chicken. Try offering honey mustard sauce, BBQ sauce, ranch dressing, mayo, Thousand Island dressing, or ketchup. The first time children try these condiments, we suggest just a tiny taste on a finger to see if they like the flavor.

Chocolate pudding

Level I

- Chocolate pudding can be offered with whipped cream or a cherry on top. These are new tastes in the context of a familiar flavor.
- Chocolate pie may be tolerated, or try offering another chocolate pastry.

Level II

- Chocolate sundaes or milk shakes may be tolerated. May be able to introduce other fruit flavors via ice cream using banana splits or sundaes. Nuts or crushed candies can be added as tolerated. These are fun "talk about food" activities that should be enjoyable and nonthreatening.
- Try offering chocolate fondue. If this is accepted, offer fruits to dip in the chocolate.

Breads

- Cheez-Its
- Goldfish crackers
- Doritos
- Try a variety of cheese-flavored crackers and chips. You can offer new flavors by offering a variety of these types of foods. Do not be concerned about the nutritional value of the foods at this time. Flavor is expanded prior to texture. (For instance, try Cool Ranch Doritos, Chicken in a Biscuit crackers, all flavors of Doritos,

Cheetos, Funyuns, flavored chips [cheddar, salt and vinegar, or BBQ]) since Melissa seems to prefer strong flavors.

Waffles and Pancakes

- Try frozen waffles or use a waffle iron or electric skillet for pancakes. (She is seeking a consistent texture with these foods and may prefer frozen because they are more consistent in texture and flavor than homemade.)
- Add pureed fruit to homemade pancakes as tolerated.
- Sprinkle with powdered sugar (light dusting).
- Peanut butter may be added in small amounts.
- Dip in maple syrup as tolerated.
- Try fruit syrups such as blueberry syrup.
- Crepes may also be accepted.

Pasta/Rice

- Pasta with butter and cheese
- Try a variety of pastas (bow tie, spiral, shells, angel hair, linguine) with butter and cheese.
- Add a tiny amount (½ Tbsp) of shredded chicken patty or nuggets to the pasta. Don't surprise her with it; instead talk to her about the chicken. Make her part of preparing meals.
- Gradually work in small amounts (1 tsp) of Alfredo or marinara sauce as tolerated.

Spreads

- Peanut butter (smooth)
- Try mini bagels with peanut butter. Peanut butter can be added to a variety of breads and crackers, and later on apple slices, celery sticks.
- Ritz Bits can be offered in peanut butter or cheddar flavors.
- Mix a small amount of honey, fruit preserve, or jelly in with peanut butter.
- Offer peanut butter cookies.

FOOD CHAINING AT DAY CARE OR SCHOOL

When your child is on a feeding program, it's vital that all of his caregivers are aware of the program and carry through with the recommendations to the best of their ability. Ask your child's occupational therapist, speech therapist, and dietitian if you can sign consent for communication between them and the day care or school. Ask if they will visit your child's day care or school to discuss the recommendations with the necessary professionals and show them how to support the program. If a visit is not possible, videotape your child in day care or school for the therapists so they can observe the environment, techniques, foods, and behavioral interventions being used. It's also helpful to have the therapists give you written recommendations to provide to the school or day care. If you don't provide your child's snack and meals, get a copy of the day care or school's daily snack and lunch menu so you can be include them as goal foods for your child to work toward.

SCHOOL

If your school-age child is overwhelmed by the cafeteria experience, whether it be the noise, lights, smells, food, number of children, or some combination thereof, a smaller, more controlled environment may be necessary. A "lunch bunch" can be formed with other children who are affected by distractions in the lunchroom or have other issues which may benefit from the modified lunch experience. Remember, it's important that your child have the opportunity for social experiences during lunch and snack time, so he should never be isolated. Here are some ideas to help your child at school:

- Select a seat for your child in the cafeteria where distractions are at a minimum (if possible).
- Go to the school and have lunch with your child in the cafeteria one day. This will give you a better idea of factors that may be impacting your child.
- Have an ongoing discussion with the person who oversees the lunchroom. It may be necessary for her to check in with your child more frequently during lunch to observe him and determine if he is eating his lunch. The lunchroom supervisor may be willing to check off on a checklist the foods that your child consumes during each lunch. Remember: Just because the lunch box comes home empty does not mean that everything was eaten. Children trade, give away, or throw away their lunches frequently.
- If your child requires special food adaptations such as a pureed diet, talk with the lunchroom supervisor to determine what modifications can be made. She may be able to store foods for your child in a refrigerator each morning to preserve the quality of the food (versus a cold pack in a lunch box). She may also be able to assist you with warming foods that have been sent from home. The school may require you to obtain a note from your

pediatrician to document the need for the special requests you are making.

- If you pack your child's lunch, rotate the foods in his lunch box that your child will eat. If the same foods are packed each day, your child is likely to reject those foods sometime in the near future. If you are working on a food chain to expand your child's restricted diet, you can place a new food item that has been successful at home, but use caution placing in the lunch box a novel food that your child is not likely to eat.

A FINAL NOTE

Your child's food-chaining program can be very successful if all the steps are completed and all your family members agree to follow the program. It isn't easy at first, and it takes time and effort, but it's worth it. The most important advice we can give you is not to rush or push your child in the beginning stages of chaining. Children can sense our anxiety at meals. Anxiety and stress are your greatest enemies in this process. Anxiety will reduce your child's appetite. Tension in your child's body can affect his swallow. If your child feels "safe" at snacks and meals, he may start to explore food on his own, and he'll be much more open to eating.

We also encourage you to remain consistent with the program, even on days when your child refuses everything and you want to throw in the towel. Your child will have good days and bad days on the program, but if you remain on track, he'll make it through. If you are feeling overwhelmed, your child may need more direct intervention from his feeding team. Don't be afraid to express your feelings and frustrations to them. An experienced team that is sensitive to your child's emotional, sensory, behavioral, and physical needs will be able to guide you through the highs and lows of the program. In the end, meals in your home will become what they should be: a pleasant and social part of family life.

CHAPTER 7

Pre-Chaining: A Precautionary Care Program for Infants

Ana and Bill's daughter Emma was born full-term but with an incomplete esophagus. The surgeons planned to connect the esophagus to the stomach in approximately two to three months, but in the meantime, a tube was placed into her stomach so she could be fed. Ana and Bill were upset that Emma would not be eating for several months and were afraid that she would forget how to suck and swallow. They were also afraid that Emma would never eat with her mouth and would need the feeding tube forever. Emma's speech therapist created a pre-chaining program for her to develop and preserve the oral skills and sensitivities that she needs to eat successfully by mouth. Emma was offered a paci-

fier during the tube feedings and the pacifier was dipped in formula several times a day so she could taste the flavor of the formula. After Emma had recovered from her surgery, her doctor allowed her to eat by mouth, and she did very well.

WHILE MANY CHILDREN have feeding disorders that only become evident over time, there are others who are born with medical conditions that prevent them from feeding properly from the get-go. For instance, extremely premature babies or infants who are diagnosed with **seizure disorder**, fine or gross motor delays, dysphagia, cardiac problems, lung problems, **cleft lip, cleft palate, tracheoesophageal fistula**, and certain genetic disorders are often unable to breast- or bottle-feed. There are still other babies who have no diagnosed medical conditions but show very early signs of feeding aversion, such as refusing the breast or bottle, gagging on baby food, crying during spoon feedings, or a general negative response to feedings. These types of problems have huge repercussions on feeding, because they can prevent children from developing the foundational feeding skills they need to learn to eat successfully in the future.

That's where pre-chaining comes in. Pre-chaining is a therapeutic technique designed to prevent infants (age birth through one year) who show early signs of a feeding problem from developing a full-blown feeding disorder. We call the technique "pre-chaining" because we're trying to avoid food chaining by nipping early feeding problems in the bud. If your infant has any of the following conditions or complications, pre-chaining can help:

- a feeding tube
- a history of a brain injury such as seizures, cerebral palsy, or bleeding in the brain
- a medical diagnosis that impacts feeding such as cleft lip, cleft palate, or heart or lung problems
- signs of feeding refusal such as crying, turning her head away from the bottle, gagging, or vomiting when food or liquid is offered

Pre-chaining was designed for infants up to one year of age, but the technique can also help older children with a history of brain injury, a medical diagnosis that affects eating, and kids on long-term or permanent feeding tubes (see box on page 229 for more information). If your child has one of these conditions or complications, talk to your doctor about whether pre-chaining might work for her.

WHAT IS PRE-CHAINING?

There is a very small window of opportunity for a baby to develop foundational feeding skills during the first year of life. If this critical period is missed due to a medical condition or an early feeding aversion, it becomes difficult for a child to learn these skills and avoid a feeding disorder. A pre-chaining program focuses on helping an infant develop her oral motor skills and oral sensory tolerance when she can't eat normally.

For instance, if your baby is being tube-fed, she is not using the muscles and structures of her mouth during feeding. This will prevent her from developing the oral motor skills she needs to master the next developmental step, which is eating from a spoon. She will also not learn to tolerate the sensation of food or liquid in her mouth, which can lead to sensory problems. Pre-chaining shows you how to mimic the experiences that a typically developing baby would have when learning to eat in a way that is specifically designed to treat the medical or swallowing difficulties that your child has. This way your baby can develop feeding skills at the proper time and rate so she won't fall behind developmentally and develop feeding problems later on.

Pre-chaining is not about getting your baby to eat—it's about making sure she develops the skills she needs to eat. While liquids and foods are usually part of the program, they are used as tools for teaching and learning, not for nutritional purposes.

Pre-chaining also focuses on oral care for maintaining the health of your baby's teeth. Many kids with feeding problems are very resistant to oral care and refuse to brush their teeth (or have them brushed), or need their parents to hold them down during dentist appointments. They can develop gingivitis and other oral care problems. Gum massage and biting and chewing on teether toys helps provide input deep into the gums where baby teeth and future teeth are hiding and helps babies become more tolerant of oral care.

PRE-CHAINING FOR OLDER KIDS

Pre-chaining was designed for infants from birth through age one, but the technique has also proven beneficial to older kids with medical or swallowing conditions that prevent them from possibly ever being able to meet their nutritional needs through oral feedings alone. In these cases, pre-chaining programs are designed to preserve sensation in and around the mouth so your child can tolerate having her teeth brushed or cared for in some way. The programs are also designed to maximize the potential that your child could have a taste of icing or ice cream at her birthday or participate in Thanksgiving dinner by having a taste of gravy.

CAN YOUR CHILD BENEFIT?

Any infant with a medical condition that interferes with feeding or who shows negative signs during feedings can benefit from a pre-chaining program. In fact, if your baby has one of the conditions we mention above or is showing early signs of feeding aversion, we encourage you to make an appointment with her pediatrician to discuss the situation. It's not unusual for parents of infants with medical conditions to be so focused on managing the condition that they don't think about how feeding may be affected. Even if they do recognize their child may have a feeding problem, a medical condition diagnosis can be so devastating that addressing yet another issue seems too overwhelming. It's important to remember that making sure your child gets optimal nutrition can only improve her medical condition. (Do note that a feeding team must have the permission of your child's pediatrician before beginning a pre-chaining program.)

HOW PRE-CHAINING WORKS

As with a food-chaining program, the first thing you need to do is take your child to her pediatrician for a checkup to uncover any medical problems and to discuss your feeding concerns. It's important to do this as soon as you can after suspecting your child has feeding issues, as the first year is a critical time for learning foundational feeding skills. Your pediatrician will likely refer you to a registered dietitian, both to assess your baby's nutritional status and to assist with implementing tube feedings, if necessary. From there, she will need to be examined by an occupational therapist and a speech therapist. These two therapists are the key players in a pre-chaining program. You will work closely with them to set goals for your baby suited to her specific needs. They will design a six-month or one-year program for her and work with you to achieve these goals. Once you and the therapists have worked out a treatment program, the therapists will contact your baby's pediatrician so he can review and sign off on it.

A typical pre-chaining program begins with your offering your infant "therapeutic tastes" several times a day. Every two to four hours, just like a typical oral feeding schedule for a baby, you'll seat your baby on your lap or in a high chair and offer her a pacifier dipped in breast milk or formula. If your baby is being tube-fed, you should do this at the same time the tube feedings are given so she can associate the experience with hunger and satiety and have the chance to regularly use the muscles of her face to suck. It's important for the therapists to closely monitor the therapeutic tastes you give your baby, because if you offer her too much too soon, she could become ill or develop pneumonia. The therapists will start your baby on the program and then allow you to give tastes once or twice a day until they determine it's safe for you to increase the amount and/or frequency of tastes.

Next the team will target chewing and biting. (However, if your baby is struggling, the next step is to offer her therapeutic tastes of pureed foods on her pacifier.) They will likely have you coat a Nuk brush (a pliable plastic brush with bristles around all sides on one end) or Thera-Band tubing (a piece of therapeutic latex-free tubing that looks like a green bean) with pureed foods to help your baby work on biting, chewing, and swallowing flavored saliva. Your baby's swallow will probably be monitored through a series of modified barium swallow studies (see chapter 3 for more information on this study), which will help the team determine how much progress she's making and judge when to increase the amount of food she can take orally. These decisions are usually made jointly by every health-care professional treating your child, not just the core members of her feeding team. So if your child has medical problems that require her to see any specialists, such as a pulmonologist or an ear, nose, and throat doctor, they will be involved in the decision-making process. Your baby will typically see the speech and occupational therapists for treatment sessions once or twice a week for the duration of her program.

PARENT PARTICIPATION IS KEY

Your participation is absolutely vital to the success of your baby's pre-chaining program. In fact, it's a serious commitment for everyone involved. You must be very careful not to give your baby more food or liquid than she can safely swallow. You must be able to understand and be on constant lookout for signs of aspiration. You must also secure the support and cooperation of every single person who participates in the care of your baby, from your partner to the grandparents to day care providers. You will all need to be trained on the mechanics of swallowing, the nature of swallowing and feeding problems, and dysphagia. All caregivers must follow to the letter the instructions given by the therapist guiding the program and report their impressions as they carry them out. It's crucial that no one stray from the program and, for instance, try to offer your infant more formula or larger bites of food than recommended. This can cause problems for your baby and in certain instances even be life-threatening.

THE FOUNDATIONAL FEEDING SKILLS

The feeding skills your baby learns during her first year of life are called foundational feeding skills because they are the skills upon which all other feeding skills are built. Foundational feeding skills are vital to your baby's successful eating in the future, and pre-chaining helps ensure that she learns them

WHAT IS SILENT ASPIRATION?

When you take a sip of a drink and it goes down the "wrong pipe," your body goes on full alert. You immediately start to cough, which is your body's way of protecting your delicate airway. Your body is trying to close off your airway so no more liquid can enter. Your eyes will water and it will take you a little while to recover. Your cough will also let others know you just aspirated.

When a baby has a swallowing disorder, her sensory receptors in the throat and the airway don't register that something has gone down the wrong pipe. She won't cough and her eyes won't water because her body is not alerted and her protective responses are not triggered. So if pureed food or liquid goes into the larynx or the trachea, the baby silently aspirates. Some children who suffer from silent aspiration have frequent colds or congestion that increases with feeding, or they limit their liquids (they drink a few ounces and stop because they feel something is not right). Silent aspiration is very dangerous and it can be quite difficult to identify. A doctor listening to your child's chest with a stethoscope can't detect silent aspiration. It does not show up on a typical chest X-ray. Only a modified barium swallow study can reveal what is going on. Repeat aspiration can scar a child's lung tissue and may cause her to develop severe and even life-threatening aspiration pneumonia. The best thing you can do is to keep a log of your concerns and your child's symptoms as they occur and show it to her pediatrician. We've seen parents have more success getting their physicians to listen when they can discuss how many times in a day something is happening. ("On Friday, my baby had a choking episode after drinking one ounce during three of her six feedings.")

when she can't or won't eat orally. Here's a quick overview of the key skills your baby needs to master:

- The suck/swallow/breathe sequence
- Swallowing secretions and saliva
- Integration of the tongue protrusion reflex
- Tolerating objects in the mouth
- Grooving or cupping the tongue around a pacifier or bottle nipple
- Biting on teethers
- Tolerating textured teethers
- Sucking and swallowing liquid
- Sucking baby food off a spoon
- More sophisticated tongue movements for finger and table foods
- Hand-to-mouth skills for self-feeding
- Biting a small solid

DID YOU KNOW?

When a baby chews on her hands in early infancy (birth to four months) or puts toys in her mouth (4 months to 12 months), she is actually preparing herself to learn the skills necessary to spoon-feed baby food and tolerate the different textures of table foods. If your baby is unable to get her hands or toys to her mouth because of a delay in motor development, you should help her do it. This will help keep her oral motor and oral sensory skills developing properly.

CREATING SENSORY EXPERIENCES WITH PRE-CHAINING

When developing a pre-chaining program for a baby, we think about the sensory experiences she would have while eating during the first year of her life and try to mimic them as closely as possible. In essence, we're looking for ways to stimulate a baby's senses without her actually having to eat anything. As you know from chapter 4, our senses are heavily involved in the act of eating. Below we detail the ways in which a pre-chaining program helps create sensory experiences for your baby to keep her on track developmentally. (We discuss smell, touch, and taste specifically because they are part of every baby's pre-chaining program. However, pre-chaining programs can certainly be created for babies with hearing and vision problems, as well.)

SMELL

The sense of smell is an important part of feeding because it helps your baby learn about food, tolerate it, and eventually enjoy it. An older infant who is not eating by mouth does not have the opportunity to smell foods, and therefore is not learning these crucial skills. Part of your baby's pre-chaining program would likely involve exposing her to the smell of food being cooked and eaten by others so she will recognize and be more apt to accept foods when the time comes for her to try them. You can do this by having her in the kitchen with you while you cook food for your family. You should also seat your baby at the table while the rest of the family is eating meals. It's a good opportunity for her to smell and learn about food even if she's not eating herself.

If you have a younger baby who is not bottle- or breast-feeding, your pre-chaining program might direct you to dip your finger in the breast milk or formula and touch her face during tube feeding so she can smell the milk on your hand.

TOUCH

Your baby needs to tolerate touch for several reasons. Touch is important to the development of your baby's tactile system (see chapter 4 for more information on the tactile system). Touch is important to the development of a close bond between you and your baby. Your baby must be able to tolerate the touch of foods and liquids on her hands to be able to interact with it. Your baby must also tolerate being touched on her face because you will need to be able to implement oral exercises to the cheeks, lips, tongue, and jaw as directed by her therapist.

The occupational therapist will design a program to help your baby learn to tolerate touch and will supervise her progress closely. She will determine the best holding techniques for both parents, as men and women have very different bodies. The therapist will also create sensory preparation programs to implement with your baby before a feeding and at different times during the day, such as transitioning to sleep, tolerating a bath, sitting in a car seat, and so forth.

Your baby may not tolerate your touch well at first, especially touches to her face. Many infants who have been in the hospital frequently have had unpleasant procedures done that involve the face, such as placement of a vent tube to help them breathe or placement of feeding tubes through the nose and mouth. A touch to their faces makes them think that something bad is going to happen. You can tell if your baby doesn't like to be touched on the face if she tenses up, grimaces, or gags, or if her breathing or color changes. If she starts to cry, she's had too much. If this is the case for you, find the level on your baby's body where she can tolerate being touched and *slowly* work your way up to her mouth as she becomes more tolerant. The goal is to get your baby to the point where she can easily tolerate being touched in and around her mouth. With some babies, tolerance of touch begins at their feet, so you may have to start there.

Pacifiers are also used to help babies become tolerant to touch in and around their mouths. Pacifiers are important because they help babies develop the skill of sucking, a foundational feeding skill, and they prepare babies to accept the nipple, spoon, and sippy cup. Babies need to be able to suck in order to extract liquid from a nipple, clear a pureed food from a spoon, and drink from a cup. Pre-chaining programs typically include specific pacifier programs, which we describe on page 239, that are designed to work on babies' sucking skills.

Most, if not all, pre-chaining programs will pair tube feedings with oral touch exercises or pacifiers to help your baby connect the feeling of fullness she gets after a tube feeding with stimulation of her mouth. Some programs will also introduce toys or feeding objects to be used as mouthing toys. A soft spoon can be used as a mouthing toy to help your baby become comfortable with its texture and presence even before any tastes are presented on it. You can give your baby the lid from a sippy cup to mouth and bite before giving her liquid to drink. Textured toys of this nature help desensitize your baby's mouth, move back the gag response, and prepare her for the texture of table foods.

TASTE

If your baby is tolerating touch to her mouth without an aversive response, it's time to work on her tolerance of taste. (Remember, we are not using foods and liquids to meet nutritional needs. We are using them to prepare and desensitize your baby's mouth.) Again, your pediatrician must approve any tastes of liquid or foods for your baby. To begin, try putting a few drops of breast milk or formula on your baby's pacifier or teether. This sounds like a very small amount, but all you want to do is add some flavor to her saliva and provide a hint of taste. You should do this while your baby is being tube-fed so she connects the taste with the feeling of fullness she's getting from the tube feeding.

When your baby reaches the age of four to six months, you can begin offering tastes of baby cereal and baby foods by applying a light film to a teether, pacifier, or soft spoon. Be sure to offer tastes from all the flavor families, including vegetables, fruits, meats, and desserts. As with any infant starting on baby food, you must systematically offer your baby tastes of one food at a time for a period to three to five days to make sure she doesn't have a food-related allergy or reaction.

At the age of 9 to 12 months, during the time that infants typically transition from baby food to table food, you can puree a small amount of your table foods and apply a light film to your baby's pacifier or spoon to provide her with an increased range of flavored foods.

PACIFIER PROGRAMS IN PRE-CHAINING

As we mentioned earlier, it's quite common for a pacifier program to be part of the larger pre-chaining program created for your baby. Pacifiers can be very beneficial for babies, especially if they are being tube-fed. They encourage the act of sucking, which helps babies develop their oral motor skills. Pacifiers prompt babies to swallow secretions, which aids in digestion, helps break fat down more quickly, and helps babies gain weight at an increased rate. A pacifier can also calm your baby, which makes her more receptive to learning and accepting sensory experiences.

USING A PACIFIER IN PRE-CHAINING

A pacifier serves many purposes in a pre-chaining program. The therapist may have you apply firm but gentle downward pressure on the pacifier two or three times in succession to help encourage tongue grooving. You may also use a technique called tractioning, where you pull gently on the pacifier while your baby is sucking on it, as if you are trying to pull it out of her mouth. Tractioning will help strengthen the suck and improve the muscles of your baby's lips so he can create a firm seal around the nipple. Tractioning is typically performed two or three times, twice in a row, twice a day. The therapist may have you apply firm pressure to your baby's palate with the pacifier to desensitize her palate. These exercises must all be learned under the supervision of your baby's therapist before you try them at home.

THE TRUTH ABOUT NIPPLE CONFUSION

There are many theories out there about "nipple confusion" and how it affects babies, most of which are untrue. Medical research shows that there are two types of nipple confusion, so here's the truth about this widely debated term.

The first type of nipple confusion describes an infant who has trouble latching on to the breast and sucking milk out properly after she has been offered a bottle. This type of nipple confusion most commonly occurs when a bottle is introduced to the baby before breast-feeding has been successfully established. It's usually caused by the difference in the flow rate between the breast and the bottle. Babies have to do very little sucking to extract milk from a bottle, especially if the bottle's flow rate is too advanced for the baby, but they must suck hard to extract milk from a breast, so bottle-feeding is much easier.

Sometimes this type of nipple confusion is caused by a sensory issue—the baby prefers the bottle because she seeks something firm in her mouth to cue her to begin sucking. This baby is successful at bottle-feeding but has difficulty breast-feeding.

The second type of nipple confusion describes an older infant who is proficient at breast-feeding and then refuses to accept a bottle. This is really "bottle refusal" instead of nipple confusion. This second type of nipple confusion is also used in reference to babies who begin to refuse the breast after accepting a bottle, but this type of refusal may actually be caused by decreased maternal milk supply or a lack of interest in nursing that comes with age.

INTRODUCING LIQUIDS IN PRE-CHAINING

After your baby's pacifier program has been firmly established, the next step is to introduce her to liquids. (Your baby should not be started on liquids without the approval of her pediatrician and a complete swallowing evaluation to make sure she is ready for this step.) This must be done in a slow and systematic way, so you can monitor your baby closely and know immediately what is successful and when problems occur. Here is the typical progression for introducing liquids in a prechaining program:

1. First, you will dip your baby's pacifier in breast milk or formula and let her suck on it.
2. Next you will inject tiny amounts of breast milk or formula from an eyedropper or syringe around the sides of the pacifier as your baby sucks on it.
3. The last step is to offer your baby small but controlled amounts of breast milk or formula that she will actually swallow.

The therapist may recommend something called a Hazelbaker FingerFeeder or Supplemental Nursing System to help with the third phase of introducing liquids. These are devices that have a holding reservoir for liquid and a small tube to deliver the liquid. They can be taped to either your finger or your baby's pacifier and deliver small, controlled amounts of liquid in a continuous flow, which encourages your baby to practice her suck/swallow/breathe skills (see chapter 4 for more information on the suck/swallow/breathe sequence). Alternatively, the therapist may have you deliver liquids to your baby with a pacifier and syringe. Once your baby is tolerating successive suck/swallow/breathe sequences in this manner, it's time to begin offering liquids through a nipple.

Our feeding team often recommends the Munchkin Medicator feeder with an alternative nipple, as the Munchkin comes with a fast-flow nipple intended for thick, syrupy medication and is not appropriate for formula or breast milk when small therapeutic amounts of oral feedings are appropriate.

When drinking from a bottle, your baby must be able to safely suck the liquid from the nipple, swallow it, and then breathe (the suck/swallow/breathe sequence), so we recommend you start with a slow-flow nipple regardless of your baby's age. Nipples are typically packaged as stages I, II, and III—stage I nipples are slow flow, stage II nipples are medium flow, and stage III nipples are fast flow. Since pre-chaining focuses on establishing the foundational feeding skills upon which all feeding skills are built, the focus is not on *how much* liquid your baby consumes, but on *how well* even a small amount of liquid is accepted. Keep in mind that you may need to try more than one nipple before you find the right one for your baby.

Your baby's therapists will closely monitor this process and help you settle on the proper nipple for your baby. They will also instruct you on how to read your baby's cues that things are not right and to judge when to try therapeutic feeds or regular bottle feeds throughout the day.

USING A SPOON IN PRE-CHAINING

In the developmental feeding progression, spoon-feeding and baby food is introduced to babies at around six months of age. Even if your baby is not yet demonstrating the skills necessary to begin spoon-feeding, we recommend you give her a spoon to mouth and bite so she can begin to establish the correct tongue and lip movements around the spoon. This is a great exercise because it allows your baby to become familiar with a spoon without having to eat any food. When the time comes to begin spoon-feeding, she will be well on her way to mastering the skill. If your baby has shown that she can swallow well and tolerate tastes of breast milk or formula, you can apply a very light film of baby food on the spoon and let your baby mouth it. This activity will combine obtaining the skills of spoon presentation with the tolerance of flavor. We usually recommend the Sassy or Gerber Soft Bite spoons, but it's important to note that every baby is unique and your therapist may have a different recommendation.

USING A CUP IN PRE-CHAINING

Sippy cups are typically introduced to babies at six months of age, but it's not a hard-and-fast rule. Babies with oral motor skill problems, for example, should not be given sippy cups with liquid in them until they demonstrate they are ready for it. Even if your child is not ready to drink liquids from a sippy cup, it's a good idea to give her one to mouth and bite to help her become familiar with it. You could even just give her the lid of a sippy cup, as the spout is the part we want her to get used to mouthing. After she gets used to the sippy cup, dip the spout in breast milk, formula, or juice and let your baby mouth it to become familiar with the feel and taste of the liquid that will typically be in the cup.

> **DID YOU KNOW?**
>
> There is no research that supports the theory that using a pacifier with a preterm infant interferes with breast-feeding.

As you can see, feeding is a complex and very challenging process that relies on the split-second precision timing of a swallow to protect the airway. Some children struggle with liquids over the long term but can eat purees and soft foods safely. Some children are never able to progress beyond therapeutic tastes, but flavorful tastes of foods and/or liquids are still very satisfying for them. If your child needs help learning her foundational feeding skills, remember to be patient—it can take time for your baby to develop the skills she needs to eat food by mouth safely, even in small amounts. Never do more than what her health-care practitioners recommend. Keeping your baby safe and healthy is the number one priority.

CHAPTER 8

Special Chains for Children with Special Needs

Six-year-old Kelsey was born with a cleft lip and palate, and feedings were difficult for her from the beginning. She had trouble bottle-feeding, so her parents, Elise and Noah, fed her with a squeeze bottle made for children with a cleft palate. At times she would cough when taking her bottle. When she started baby food, she didn't seem to swallow it like other babies do. She pressed her tongue up to the roof of her mouth. Since she had a cleft, Elise and Noah could see some of the food coming out through her nose. They noticed that she did not have as much food come out through her nose when it was thicker, but when it did happen, it was difficult to clear from her nostrils.

To help solve this problem, Kelsey's speech therapist developed an oral motor program to improve her ability to move food back properly for swallowing. The therapist also developed food chains for her to work on her feeding skills and give her more sensory input at meals. The therapist reduced the size of each bite of food and positioned Kelsey with additional support in her high chair. Through food chaining, Elise and Noah changed their feeding technique and learned that Kelsey ate better when foods were very flavorful. As she progressed through the chains, Kelsey began making up her own combinations of strong-flavored foods. For example, she would dip her green beans in applesauce and her bananas in ketchup. She made some crazy combinations, but they appealed to her and she ate more at meals. Prior to using food chaining, all the foods they'd offered Kelsey were very bland. Her parents thought back a month earlier to when they were giving Kelsey regular unflavored oatmeal and very large bites of food, and they finally understood why she hadn't been eating well.

IT'S VERY EASY to become blinded by the "labels" that are placed on our kids, especially kids with special needs. Children with special needs are still just kids, and they often have more than one medical problem if we look beyond the major diagnosis of "autism" or "Down syndrome." As therapists and medical professionals, we must do our very best to remove the blinders and keep looking. The fact is that many children with special needs also struggle with feeding problems, and they must be addressed.

If your child has special care needs, you may be thinking, "I have so many things to worry about, I can't take this on, too." Your life may consist of one medical or therapy appointment after another. You may lie awake at night feeling afraid for your child, worrying about schools and finding the right treatment programs, medications, and doctors for him. You may wonder how your child's life will turn out, and what would happen to him if something happened to you. The fatigue, stress, and pain you feel may be crippling at times. We won't pretend that food chaining is easy, but we can tell you that it's worth the extra effort. Good nutrition is at the heart of our good health, and making sure your child is getting optimal nutrition will benefit him in every aspect of his life. We have seen children with special needs thrive and make huge gains in their treatment after their feeding problems have been addressed with food chaining. They are well hydrated, their lungs are protected from aspiration and respiratory infections, they sleep better, and food becomes something they enjoy instead of dread.

Depending on your child's condition, his feeding team may recommend a feeding tube and break your heart. But remember this: There is a reason that over 90 percent of parents report that they are happy they decided to place a gastrostomy tube (g-tube)—they see improvement in their children. A feeding tube does not spell the end of feeding by mouth for most children. With the right treatment program, he may still be able to eat a small amount of food by mouth, and eating will become a pleasurable experience for him instead of a chore. For some children, the g-tube is a stepping stone to eating by mouth. It depends on the child and the medical condition.

In this chapter, you will hear from Alicia Hart. Her son Ewan has autism, but he is so much more than the "autism." He is a bright light in the world with a great big soul. He loves everyone around him and it costs him dearly to do so. His sensory system batters him as he tries to be in this world with all its noises, sounds, and smells. When we met Ewan, he was a very selective eater. When we looked beyond his autism, we discovered that he also had eosinophilic esophagitis and dysphagia, and we were concerned that he had enlarged tonsils and adenoids that affected his swallowing. If we had just stopped at "autism," we would have failed Ewan, and his food-chaining program would have failed as well.

When you reach the sample food chains in this chapter, you'll see that we look at every aspect of a child's life in these programs, from how he is transported to school to how he sleeps at night. Stress and anxiety affect appetite, and that's a big issue for kids with special needs. Our goal is to create a world that protects them from sensory overload yet allows them to become more tolerant of sensory input over the course of treatment.

AUTISM

One in 150 children is diagnosed with autism, making it more common than pediatric cancer, diabetes, and AIDS combined. There's still a lot we don't know about the condition, but we do know that it impairs a child's ability to communicate and relate to others. Many kids with autism exhibit rigid or repetitive behaviors, such as obsessively arranging objects or following very specific routines. The symptoms affect every child differently, and can range from very mild to quite severe.

Feeding is also typically a problem for autistic kids, though it is not always recognized due to the multitude of other concerns involved in caring for them. They often have global sensory issues and react negatively to textures, tastes, and smells. Many children with autism eat in ways that people perceive as strange. They may pick apart their food: taking the cheese off their pizza, then eating the bread. If you give them a cheeseburger, they may eat the cheese, hamburger, and bun separately. Sometimes they will peel the breading off chicken nuggets and eat that separately from the chicken.

Many of the autistic children we see eat just a few foods with a uniform texture, such as crackers and chips or McDonald's chicken nuggets, and they will not accept substitutes easily. Many autistic children also prefer to drink rather than eat, or to drink or eat in order to regulate their sensory system. Children with autism don't always associate hunger with eating, and as adults they often forget to eat. A feeding program for an autistic child should involve teaching him that he needs to eat a certain number of times each day and associating eating with his daily routine.

Getting children with autism to eat can be difficult, but since much of their problem is sensory in nature, it is possible to develop effective feeding programs for children on the spectrum.

THE AUTISM LIFE
ALICIA HART, MOTHER OF FOUR-YEAR-OLD EWAN

When I hear the word *autism,* two concepts come to mind: perspective and instinct. I think of perspective because it is what I need to understand my four-year-old son Ewan. Ewan has autistic spectrum disorder, which affects the way he understands the world, learns new things, and interacts with others. In a sense, Ewan spends much of his time in his own world, a world that is completely separate from mine. I am Ewan's guide to my world, the "neurotypical" world, and in order to be a good guide I need to see his perspective as often as I try to teach him mine.

I think of instinct because I must constantly remind myself that Ewan's instincts are not the same as other children's. Neurotypical children, or children without autism, are born with certain instincts. For instance, an infant instinctually knows to root for a nipple and food. An infant instinctively knows how to mold his body to the shape of his mother when she holds him. An infant is instinctively interested in his mother's face and watches her eyes, lips, and expressions. He will even instinctively respond to that first bit of "baby talk." A toddler is instinctively interested in what his parents are eating and reaches for it with gusto. All of these instincts are often missing in a child with autism. An autistic child *can* learn, but sometimes the simplest acts need to be broken down for him and taught explicitly.

There are many different degrees of autism (hence the "spectrum"). Your child may have only a few quirks, or he may need intense support and accommodations to learn and grow in this world.

Either way, eating and mealtimes often become part of the daily struggle between what you want as a parent and what your autistic child can handle.

I vividly remember the meal that was my breaking point with Ewan, what made me decide to seek help from Cheri and the rest of the feeding team. My husband had made this wonderful dinner (shrimp creole) that smelled amazing. My two-year-old sat at the table and began scooping up rice and popping it into his mouth without hesitation. But Ewan could barely stand to be in the same house with us. He cried just because we asked him to sit with us at the table. I thought, *How hard can this really be?* I lost whatever perspective I had on his sensory issues and his lack of communication skills and decided that *he was going to try this food.* When Ewan got to the point where he was starting to hyperventilate and shake like a leaf because he was crying so hard, my husband put his hand on my arm and said, "He can't do it. He just can't." We both knew then that this was something that we couldn't deal with on our own. We needed help.

I remember, after our first meeting with the feeding team, feeling overwhelmed. I could understand the part about slowly adding flavors, tastes, and textures into Ewan's diet through food chaining. What I didn't understand was the food education part. Why on earth did we need to teach Ewan about food? Didn't he know what food was for?

In the end it was Ewan who showed me the path to understanding, as it usually is. We happened to be watching a show about how foods are made, basic ones like milk, apples, peanut butter, and potatoes. He was fascinated and it was only then that he wanted to try these foods. He saw how they were made, he saw people eating them, and it just clicked for him. That's when I realized that Ewan *didn't* instinctively understand the purpose of food and eating, and why food education was so important to his treatment.

With help from his therapist and guidance from Cheri and the other members of the feeding team, it slowly came together for Ewan. He started to tolerate picking up foods, licking foods, tasting foods, and rating his food, and he wanted to know more about food in general. Food chaining is hard, it takes time, and progress is not made overnight, but it becomes part of your life, and it works. Your child will learn to eat as well as he can, and that's all you can ask for.

SENSORY PROCESSING DISORDER AND AUTISM

As you learned in chapter 4, our senses play an integral role in our tolerance of foods, therefore affecting our success with feeding. If your child has autism, he has a condition that affects his ability to interpret, organize, and act on sensory information. This is very important to appreciate, as his world is completely different from ours. Internally he struggles a great deal just to prepare himself for the task of eating. For example, when he sits down for a meal, his body is assaulted by sensory input from all sides. He's affected by the lights in the room, the number of people sitting at the table, the noise level in the room, the feeling of the chair beneath him, the clothing he's wearing, the aromas of food, the texture of the food when he touches it, the taste of the food when he first puts it in his mouth, and the changes that occur when he crushes the food with his teeth. A lot is happening to your child, and it's all occurring around his hands and mouth, which are highly sensitive areas.

Your child's sensory issues may also cause him to be overly sensitive to many textures of food. Many children with autism prefer foods with one particular texture that does not change when they chew it. They usually find meat, fruits, and vegetables very aversive because they have such complex textures. Children with autism are not capable of predicting the texture of a food before they bite into it, and this is particularly disturbing for them. If an autistic child bites into a food and the "food label," or the sensory properties of the food, is not what he was expecting, he may freeze with the food on his tongue. He may become so overwhelmed with sensory input that he forgets how to start the motor sequence needed to chew the food. The food is literally stuck in his mouth while his brain is flooded with competing sensory input that he doesn't know how to appropriately and automatically filter, interpret, and respond to. He responds the only way he knows how: by spitting the food out of his mouth. The parent, not understanding the complexity of the situation, will commonly correct the child. This negative experience may continue to affect him for days, weeks, and even months. If the child continues to be pushed to eat foods he cannot tolerate, eating will become something that he fears and avoids to some degree.

Many children with autism are sensitive to the point where they can detect even the subtlest changes in food and easily tell one brand from another. We've had many parents ask us why their child has such a regimented eating pattern, and it all links back to how they process sensory input (see chapter 4 for an in-depth look at the sensory aspects of feeding). Children with sensory processing disorders are bombarded with sensory input that they can't process and respond to normally, and they spend much of their time feeling uncomfortable and unsafe. They are drawn to foods, routine, toys, clothing, and people that are familiar and predictable. So it makes sense that when children with autism eat a meal, they seek food that feels safe to them. Kids with autism "cope" with eating by finding and clinging to a few foods that they know how to eat with success. Sensory processing disorder can also affect your child's digestion and elimination. It can be difficult for him to understand signals from the body telling him it's time to urinate or pass a bowel movement. Some autistic children are chronically constipated, which can dampen their desire to eat. Constipation can also cause pain in the GI tract by disrupting the waves of normal movement (also known as peristalsis).

TRY NOT TO SET LIMITS

The same rigidity that autistic children show in their selective eating also demonstrates their capacity to learn about food. Autistic children observe everything about their food, from the labels on the food item to the color and style of their cup, plate, or utensil, and they can distinguish between a french fry from Burger King and one from McDonald's. Children with autism *can* learn. In fact, many times these special children have truly exceptional learning abilities. Too often, we set limits for children in our own minds. We think, *He won't eat that,* and we don't offer the food. It becomes a self-fulfilling prophecy. Remember, he won't eat it if you don't offer it. .

REACTIONS TO FOOD

If your child has autism, his experiences with food may always be negative unless he is eating a food he knows well. There are a few ways an autistic child may react to food he is either uncomfortable with and/or does not want to eat:

1. He could have an immediate and uncontrollable fight-or-flight response. A fight response is aggressive. For example, your child may act hostile when offered food by throwing the plate across the room. A flight response is avoidant, meaning your child may run away from the food. A fight-or-flight response is an act of desperation on your child's part. He's attempting to withdraw immediately from the situation.

2. He may practice avoidance. This means your child recognizes that the act of eating is too much to tolerate and stops. Or he may also react with panic or anger when faced with a mealtime environment or situation. Children with autism will avoid food when they perceive daily meals as land mines full of unknown negative experiences that are unpleasant, painful, or frightening.

One of the keys to an effective feeding program is finding foods to offer your child that do not trigger these types of responses. This is done by carefully analyzing the foods your child likes, used to like, and hates. This provides us with his "eating profile." We can then begin cautiously expanding his diet knowing that changes need to be graded and gentle. To make the process more comfortable for your child, his feeding team will not alter his "anchor foods," or the foods he needs to feel secure, until much later in treatment, if at all. For some children the sight of an anchor food on a plate is comforting and cues them to begin eating. Even in small portions, anchor foods are very important to these kids.

THE GLUTEN-FREE, CASEIN-FREE DIET

There is research that suggests that foods containing gluten (the protein in wheat, oats, rye, and barley) and casein (the protein in milk products) should be avoided by autistic children as it may affect their neurological processes. Most people have the ability to break down gluten and casein proteins into peptides and further into amino acids. The opioid excess theory proposes that excess peptides from incomplete digestion of gluten and casein act as opioids and disrupt neurotransmitters in autistic children, which leads to behavioral changes. The unbroken-down peptides enter the bloodstream and create an opiate-like effect that depresses the activity of their nervous system. The theory suggests that this opiate-like effect creates a chemical dependency that causes autistic children to crave and often be unable to stop eating foods that contain gluten and casein.

We've had many families ask about this diet and want to attempt it with their children. We neither encourage nor discourage them from using it as a treatment option. At this point, the gluten-free, casein-free diet is considered experimental, and more research is necessary. We provide families with the medical facts regarding the risks and possible benefits of the diet and allow them to decide if they wish to pursue it. (You should never attempt this diet, or any treatment for that matter, without your pediatrician's approval.)

KNOW THE RISKS AND COSTS OF THIS DIET

If you do decide to try the gluten-free, casein-free diet, your child will need to avoid all gluten and casein. This puts him at risk for nutritional deficiencies, such as calcium, iron, magnesium, phosphorus, zinc, and many B vitamins. He may also be deficient in essential amino acids. Vitamin and mineral supplements are often necessary when following this diet. Children who absolutely refuse to take a vitamin are not good candidates for this diet. Neither are children with extremely selective repertoires (such as three foods) that include only foods that contain gluten and casein.

You should also weigh the costs of a gluten-free, casein-free diet before you begin. You will need to buy special food items that are often much more expensive than traditional food items. For example, regular pasta may cost five cents per ounce whereas gluten-free pasta can cost up to 26 cents per ounce. You may also have to look far and wide for the foods that you need for your child and spend a lot more time grocery shopping. Your other family members may be inconvenienced as a result of this diet. You may not be able to eat at many restaurants because your child may be exposed to gluten and casein at these locations.

GETTING STARTED

When starting a gluten-free, casein-free diet, pick a time in your child's life when he is not starting other interventions or therapies. This will enable you and your feeding team to see direct results from the diet. This diet is most often implemented for a minimum of three to six months in order to determine whether there have been any changes in your child's behavior. Be sure to have your child's feeding team get a baseline measurement of his behaviors before starting the program so that an objective measurement of change can occur after implementation.

Many families begin by eliminating casein first, as it is often easier to find acceptable alternatives to milk products such as soy or rice milk. (You should note that some of these alternatives do not contain adequate amounts of fats or proteins.) After you've gotten into the routine of avoiding casein, you can take the next step and cut out the gluten.

You must be vigilant about reading food labels when your child is on this diet, as gluten and casein can be found in many unexpected foods. For example, hot dogs or rice cakes may contain milk. Gluten may be found in things such as modified food starch, caramel coloring, and hydrolyzed or vegetable protein. Your child's gluten-free, casein-free diet should be monitored by a dietitian or pediatrician with experience in food allergies, celiac disease, or autism. These professionals can offer valuable advice on every aspect of the diet, such as how to read food labels, find specialty food items, prevent cross-contamination, and eat out as a family, to name a few.

KIDS WITH AUTISM DON'T ALWAYS EAT OUT OF HUNGER

It's not unusual for autistic children to eat or drink for reasons other than hunger. For instance, a child with autism may drink from a spill-free sip cup because he likes the feeling of resistance he receives from the valve, and the taste of juice is predictable. He's receiving oral input from the cup during the act of drinking that makes him feel calm and in control. Unfortunately, if this type of intake becomes a pattern, the child will drink until he is so full that he doesn't feel hunger anymore.

DID YOU KNOW?

Some children with autism avoid the table during meals because the multiple aromas of food, the sounds of people eating, and the appearance of what used to be a clean, clutter-free table now covered with food can make them feel anxious and overwhelmed. We treated a child who would cover his mother's mouth with his hands when she ate because he couldn't stand the sounds of her eating. Some kids become overwhelmed by the sounds they hear in their own heads when chewing food.

FOOD CHAINING WITH AUTISM

A feeding program is created for an autistic child in much the same way it is for a neurotypical child. He must be examined by his pediatrician for underlying medical conditions that could be contributing to his feeding disorder. He must also be examined by a dietitian to assess his nutritional needs, a speech therapist to assess his feeding skills, an occupational therapist to determine the exact nature of his sensory problems, and a psychologist to evaluate his behavior. Children with autism almost always need to attend occupational therapy to work on their sensory issues as well as speech therapy to sharpen their feeding skills. Occupational therapy usually comes first. We may schedule a child's liquids and meals, rotate his core foods, and add calories if he drinks milk with a small amount of Carnation Instant Breakfast or PediaSure, but not change his diet a great deal until the occupational therapist has had time to work with him. In the meantime, we typically provide "learning about food" ideas for the child and therapist to use during treatment.

Once we reach the point where the child is ready to expand his diet, we try to introduce new foods and make changes based on your child's sensory system and preferences, as we do with all food chains. We study the foods your child currently eats and make the smallest change by offering him a food that is almost identical to what he already likes. This shows your child that a little change is safe and helps him start to trust you and eating again. The feeding team will help you learn how to offer food in a systematic way and feel more confident at meals. They will build on successful eating experiences and expand the number of foods in your child's diet at his own pace.

Here are some tips to help you ensure a successful feeding program for your autistic child:

Use the food-chaining intake form. Located in appendix 3, the food-chaining intake form is designed to help you and your child's feeding team analyze the foods your child prefers, previously accepted, and rejects. Once you've located the patterns in these food items, you and the team can select one or two foods to try that your child is likely to accept. It's very important to know your child's food patterns inside and out. You and the team should quickly come to a point where you can suggest foods for his food chains without looking at his intake form. The rating scales will help you see what changes are being tolerated so you can decide on the next step.

Start slowly and be patient. When you offer your child new foods, do so slowly and stick with the food chains the feeding team has created. Do not offer your child a food you think he should eat; offer him a food you are confident he can tolerate well. Remember that these are all new routines your child is learning, so be patient with him. If you rush ahead or overwhelm him with too much change, you could sabotage his program and make him feel even more unsafe and resistant to meals.

Closely observe your child's reactions. Your observations of your child's reactions to foods are critical because they help the feeding team choose additional foods that he is likely to accept. Your observations, along with the rating scale, are what keep the food chain working for your child.

Your child will show you with his facial expressions and gestures that he doesn't like a food, but often signs of distress are very subtle. Grimaces, wide eyes, changes in breathing pattern, changes in color, splaying of fingers, shrugging of the shoulders, wiping hands on clothing, and sticking the tongue out of the mouth all indicate displeasure. You must also watch your child carefully and study how he looks when he's given a food he does enjoy. Keep track of your observations in a notebook or journal so you can easily share them with the team. The occupational therapist will be instrumental in helping you learn to read all your child's responses to food, whether they are pleasurable, neutral, or negative.

Always rate your child's reactions to new food. The rating scales are key to food chaining because they track your child's progress and help the feeding team continue to customize the program to your child's unique needs. See chapter 6 for an in-depth discussion on how to use the rating scales. Be sure to track your ratings on a calendar or notepad to share with the feeding team.

Give your child time to explore food. The process of accepting a new food involves every sense and every organ. Your child needs time to explore a food visually and to be exposed to the aroma of the food before you can expect him to touch it or taste it. Touching food gives your child a great deal of information, and it's the first step in preparing his mouth for the sensation of the food. Be patient and give him as much time to explore the food as he needs.

Do not insist your child use utensils. This tip links back to the exploration of food above. Your child must be able to touch food before he can eat it. Touching food also prepares your child for the sensations he will feel inside his mouth when he takes a bite of food. This is a very important part of the feeding program. To this end, don't insist that he use utensils while eating or reprimand him for using his fingers. There will come a time in your child's program where he will begin working on utensil use, but right now it's more important that he has the opportunity to explore all of the sensory properties of the food and store this information for future use.

TEACHING KIDS WITH AUTISM ABOUT FOOD

Sometimes we have the wonderful opportunity to work with families who truly change our lives and teach us more than any institution of higher learning could possibly teach us. Alicia Hart and her son Ewan are one of those families (see "The Autism Life" box on page 249). Ewan has autistic spectrum disorder, so we developed a treatment program customized to his special needs and suggested ways Alicia could teach him about food. Teaching children with autism about food can be a challenge, but it's vital to their success at food chaining. Alicia took that information and, together with Ewan's speech pathologist Stacey Vitale, CCC/SLP, from Sarah Bush Lincoln Hospital in Mattoon, Illinois, came up with incredible learning activities for all children, but particularly those with autism. Alicia generously shares some of her tips below. Try to do a food activity with your child several times a week, either at home or in feeding therapy.

BEFORE YOU GET STARTED

The point of these activities is to provide your child with ways to explore the sensory properties of food to both teach him about food and help improve his sensory tolerance. The most effective way to teach autistic children is through active learning situations, where they participate in a process and see how things work. Most of these activities involve handling food, so make sure your child can tolerate touching the foods you are working with before using them. Keep a wet washcloth and a towel on the table by your child so he can clean and dry his hands as needed.

Sitting down for more than a minute or two can be difficult for children with autism, and your child will need to be able to sit at a table to participate in many of these activities. Work on sitting with him every day, even if he only sits for a few seconds at a time at first. This will also help increase the time he can tolerate sitting at the table at meals.

Color Coloring is a great way to learn about food. Buy a coloring book that features foods or ask your child to draw specific foods for you. You can also buy stickers of food and even food stickers that smell like food to add to the fun. Pull out a few real foods like carrots, broccoli, or cucumber for your child to touch and play with as part of his artwork.

Finger Paint Your child can use finger paint to draw foods and dip sponges in the shape of foods into paint. The sponges are especially great if your child cannot yet tolerate touching paint with his fingers. You can also use pudding or pureed fruits and vegetables as finger paints.

Do a Scavenger Hunt You can create a scavenger hunt for your child using food. Have him locate all the ingredients you need to make a recipe or hide food items around the house and offer him a prize for finding them. If your child is tolerating foods well, you could even have him take bites of the foods he finds.

Play Food Bingo You can make a bingo board using real foods, making it clear your child is not expected to eat them.

You can use Ritz Bits, baby pretzels, grapes, raisins, popcorn, cherry tomatoes, baby carrots, and little cookies. The possibilities are endless.

Count Ask your child to help you count during food-related activities. Have him count the number of plates you will need at dinner, or how many people will be eating. Talk about how many bites you are going to take of your food, how many pieces of chicken are on your plate, and how many chocolate chips are in a cookie.

Classify Foods Alicia tells us that children with autism are already classifying their food items into two categories—food they will eat and food they will never touch. In order to help your child classify foods in more productive ways, talk to your child about where foods come from. You don't need to know the scientific name for every vegetable, just point out that asparagus is a veggie and bread is a grain. Talk about which foods grow from seeds and which ones come from animals. The point is to help your child understand that foods don't just come from your refrigerator or the grocery store.

Measure Food There are lots of ways you can measure foods and get your child to engage with them. You can use the traditional measuring cup or spoon. You can add a "pinch of salt," or use an eyedropper or a turkey baster to measure liquids. If your child likes to watch water fall, you can put a liquid into one container and pour it into another over and over again.

Make Fun Food Shapes You can cut big and small slices of bread or pull cheese apart to make different-sized chunks. You can cut foods into triangles and other shapes, or use a cookie cutter to make other fun shapes out of bread, thin cheese slices (like Kraft singles), or dough.

Take a Food Field Trip Take your child to a factory to see how a particular food is made. Take him to a farm to see how plants grow, watch cows get milked, or watch eggs get collected from chickens. Go to a historical site where they churn butter by hand. Letting your child observe you prepare food is also very educational. Have him watch you make dinner and see what happens to food when it is cut, squished, blended, cooked, and frozen. This can help your child understand that food changes all the time. They can change as they grow (like grapes and raisins or plums and prunes) and they can change in terms of texture, substance, and color as they are prepared and cooked.

Play with Photos Download and print out photos of food from the Internet or cut food photos out of magazines and off packages to make collages. Ask your child to group together the foods he wants to eat for dinner one night, or give him a bunch of photos and ask him to classify them. You can even download food photos and transfer them to edible paper to decorate a cake. (There are photos available on government Web sites that are in the public domain. For instance, the USDA Web site has photos of farms, tractors, grocery stores, kids at school cafeterias, seeds, plants, and animals. There is also a link to the Food and Nutrition Service site, which has videos about healthy eating and clip art for kids.)

TEACHING YOUR CHILD THE ART OF PREDICTION

After your child has grasped the concepts of counting, classifying, measuring, and observing through the activities listed above, it's time to teach him how to predict how a food will taste and what it will feel like in his mouth. Making predictions about food is hard for autistic children because they often lack the instinct to do it. For instance, a typically developing child can predict with reasonable certainty what a carrot is going to look like, taste like, or smell like every time they come in contact with a carrot. Children with autism must be taught this skill. This is why they usually fear new foods.

To teach your child how to make predictions about food, you must talk your child through the experience of eating all kinds of food and offer as much descriptive detail about the foods as possible. Take a carrot, for example. If you tell your child that carrots grow from seeds, that they are orange and crunchy, that they can be bitter sometimes and sweet at other times (even within the same carrot), this will make sense to him. Eventually, with plenty of positive reinforcement, visual aids, and practice, your child will learn to predict what will happen when he takes a bite of a carrot.

COLIN'S FOOD-CHAINING PROGRAM

Thirteen-year-old Colin was diagnosed with autistic spectrum disorder at age six. He follows routines and produces a few single words. Colin spent several years in the foster care system before he and his three brothers were adopted by a loving family when he was nine. In foster care, he spent time in many different homes and environments, which had a negative impact on his development. His adoptive family is very motivated to help him and they have made great progress in therapy and with home programs, but they continue to struggle with meals and are worried about his nutrition.

Family Goal: To improve Colin's nutrition, provide a balanced diet, and make mealtimes less stressful.

Step 1: Medical Evaluation Colin has no medical problems, but he is undernourished. This places him at greater risk for a variety of health problems, such as illness and infection, reduced rate of growth, and developmental delays, as well as more educational and social problems.

Step 2: Nutrition Evaluation Colin's weight gain is slow and he is very small for his age. His skin is very pale. He is undernourished and he will not accept a vitamin. Colin will not accept oral nutritional supplements, and a supplemental feeding tube is not appropriate at this time because his weight gain is slow but he does not qualify as having failure to thrive. The nutritionist felt that with improvement in his food repertoire, he would improve his weight gain and nutritional status. The nutritionist suggested Scooby-Doo Fizzy Vites vitamins be crushed and added to drinks made of juice, sherbet, and a small amount of 7UP. This combination of liquids was chosen to mask the vitamin flavor and texture. His caloric intake is not optimal, which is affecting his energy level, sleep cycle, and overall nutritional status.

Step 3: Feeding Evaluation Colin's oral motor and swallowing skills are within normal limits, but he can't tolerate the sensory properties of many foods. His food selectivity is linked to his sensory processing disorder.

Steps 4 and 5: Sensory and Behavioral Evaluation Colin was observed via videotape in many different environments. This allowed the team to design a program to meet his needs at home, at school, and in the community.

> ***Sensory Observations at School and at Home*** Colin is transported to school by bus. He is on the school bus for approximately forty minutes prior to arriving at school. Riding the bus and walking down the hall full of noisy children frightens and overwhelms him. By the time Colin arrives at school and gets to his classroom, he is on full sensory overload and the day hasn't even started yet. Every day when Colin gets to school, he retreats to the corner in his classroom and wants to play with Legos. The teacher and classroom aide report many behavioral breakdowns, such as screaming and banging his head, when they try to redirect Colin to activities in the classroom after he arrives at school. When they do succeed in

redirecting him, they report that Colin is stressed out and volatile for the rest of the day.

By the time Colin goes to the cafeteria for lunch, he is having full-blown meltdowns. He covers his ears if there is too much auditory stimulation. Colin appears to tolerate one person speaking with no problem, but if several adults are talking or laughing loudly, he becomes distressed and leaves the area. The smells of perfume, cologne, and cleaning products, and the wide range of other odors around him are at times overwhelming. We cannot know what Colin experiences when he is stressed to this level. It may be painful. It may last for a very long time. He may feel something close to panic at times. We can only observe his behaviors to see what he is drawn to and what he enjoys. He likes the sound and sensation of running water over his hands in the bathroom, but does not tolerate the sound of flushing toilets.

At home, Colin assembles five-thousand-piece jigsaw puzzles and keeps himself busy with play with Legos, building blocks, and assembling toys. He has very few behavioral outbursts. This is important information for the team. Colin can tolerate the safe, quiet environment at home and is not distressed by the aromas of food preparation.

Communication and Learning Skills Colin speaks several single words, but his spoken language and understanding of language in general is very delayed. Colin learns best when someone briefly labels items or describes actions as he is touching and exploring items around him. We suggested reducing the amount of speech used in interaction with Colin, as he is sensitive to sound and can't process longer sentences. To Colin, too much language sounds like someone speaking a foreign language at a very rapid rate. In time it becomes annoying and distracting. Colin wants to interact with others, but it's very hard for him to do so. If everyone in the world would just sit still and be quiet, he could handle the auditory and visual stimulation around him. Patterns in the clothing people wear bother him. He wants his mother to wear a dark blue sweatshirt all the time. He puts his head against her and shuts out the world. His mother is fearful that he will run away from her in a store or parking lot.

Mealtime Observations at Home Colin will eat at the table at home, but he prefers to sit alone. If someone is eating close by him, he puts his hands over the person's mouth. He does not like the sounds of other people eating or chewing gum. When his mother puts new foods on the table in front of him, Colin becomes upset and anxious. We need to determine if this is a reaction to the sensory properties of the food on the table or a reaction to the table appearing different, cluttered, and out of order. Colin gets up from the table and moves away from the food. Colin's mother reports that he only wants his core food items on his plate. However, we observed that Colin is drawn to the aroma of spicy foods. He gets as close to his mother as possible when she eats foods like pizza with Italian sausage or chicken chipotle rolls. This is significant, because now we know that Colin is drawn to the pleasing aroma of spicy foods. We feel he is highly likely to accept food items with a spicy aroma given more exposure and teaching time. So we will explore meals over the course of treatment to see how Colin responds to foods that have high sensory feedback. We will also see if he is happier with serving bowls removed from the table to reduce excessive visual distraction.

Mealtime Observations at School The school cafeteria is completely overwhelming to Colin, to the point where he either has an emotional outburst or shuts down, sitting with his hands over his face, and doesn't eat. His teachers are trying to change his behavior without understanding the motivation behind it. This is Colin's way of telling us that the sounds, smells, and movement of the lunchroom are too much for him to handle.

School Environment Modifications The team focused on reducing distractions in Colin's environment throughout the day. We discussed Colin's bus route with the school and determined that if the current bus route was reversed, Colin would only have to spend 10 minutes on the bus. Colin's routine of going to the corner of his classroom to play with Legos when he arrived at school was allowed to continue as a way to help him regulate his sensory system, but the amount of time he spent playing was reduced. We suggested that Colin go to his occupational therapist in the morning before starting other activities. The occupational therapist provided alternative activities that appealed to Colin and motivated him to participate in more classroom learning activities.

During lunch, Colin went to the cafeteria with his aide and two peers before the rest of the children were taken to lunch. The cafeteria staff did not run the dishwasher while Colin was in the cafeteria. A Sleepmate was used to provide background white noise and help Colin focus on his food. A picture schedule was used at each meal. The occupational therapist modified Colin's seating so he had support to his body and under his feet while eating. A small fan was placed beside the table to help Colin tolerate the aromas in the cafeteria. In this quieter environment, Colin was able to eat a small amount of food. His intake gradually improved over time.

Step 6: The Food Chains Colin is an extremely picky eater, and 14 food items dropped from his food repertoire over the last year. He has strong flavor and texture preferences and refuses all fruits, vegetables, and meats. Colin prefers salty flavors and the bubbly input of carbonated beverages. He prefers crunchy, uniform textures and rejects mixed-texture foods.

COLIN'S CORE DIET

Accepted Foods and Liquids Colin has strong food preferences, and needs the sensory feedback he gets from crunchy, crispy, or strong-flavor foods. French fries, crackers, milk, Pepsi, and 7UP are the only foods and drinks he consistently accepts.

Team Recommendations Our team met with Colin's family, therapists, and school staff to explain his food-chaining program. We discussed how foods must be presented to Colin so he can explore them with his senses to prepare him for eating. The team explained the sensory hierarchy approach to introducing new foods (see chapter 6 for more information) and how children with autism do not have the ability to immediately evaluate the properties of a food by appearance and touch. Repeat exposures to food would be necessary. The team cautioned everyone that progress would be very slow in the beginning, but once Colin accepted a bit of variety in his diet, he would be much more likely to accept more foods in the future, with less teaching time required. Colin has gone on several food jags (see chapter 2 for more information), so we explained why they happen and offered strategies to help reduce their occurrence.

The rest of Colin's treatment program was focused on teaching him about new foods, expanding his taste and texture preferences, and improving his overall intake of food and liquid. We suggested that Colin participate in food preparation and that the family set a routine for all meals, including washing hands, setting the table, serving food to family members, and helping with cleanup. This will teach Colin how to predict what will happen at each meal and lessen his anxiety about mealtime. A picture schedule should be used to help Colin know that meals have a beginning and an end point. Colin should be offered three meals and two to three snacks each day.

Teaching about Food: Colin's teacher and therapist used snack time at school as teaching time for all the children. Colin participated in activities and gradually started tasting new foods after observing the other children eat the foods. However, he would often reject the same food if it was offered at home. His parents were told that children often eat differently in different environments, and they should keep offering Colin these foods in small portions at home without expecting him to eat them.

Therapy Referrals: Colin receives weekly speech and occupational therapy at school. We provided a feeding program for the school team to implement and consulted with them on any problems they had along the way.

COLIN'S FOOD-CHAINING PROGRAM

Food Modifications The first level of the food-chaining program included gentle modifications of accepted food items. The family and school staff used clip art, coloring pages, toy foods, and videos about food from the Cosmeo Web site (see

Resources for more information) and other teaching sites to expose Colin to new foods.

COLIN'S FOOD CHAINS

Salty, Crunchy Foods: Colin eventually accepted a variety of crackers and chips. He also accepted cheese, so we were able to move on to quesadillas and thin-crust cheese pizza.

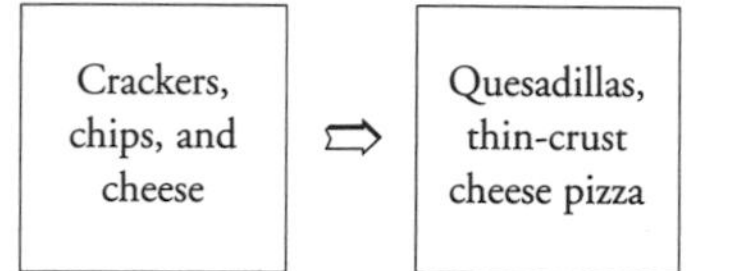

Sweet, Crunchy Foods: He accepted cinnamon twists and, later, thin-crust pastries with apple.

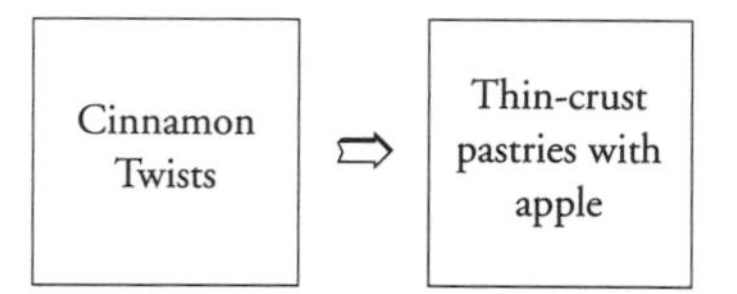

French fries: A wide variety of types and brands of french fries was explored over an eight-week period. Colin accepted store brands of frozen fast-food-style fries baked on a baking stone after repeated exposure to them. Colin was offered his preferred fries on a divided plate or tray or on a separate small plate if he wanted. The serving size was three or four new fries. Colin was resistant to changes except with french fries, and the team felt that once he accepted more variety in fries, he would be more accepting of other changes. No other modifications were made in the beginning weeks of treatment. Gradually we worked toward tolerance of preferred fries and targeted fries on the same plate. Colin's siblings broke fries into pieces, talked about fries, and modeled eating new fries to him. Colin participated in putting the new fries on a baking sheet prior to cooking. Eventually new food items were also placed on Colin's plate, solely for exposure. The family cooked small amounts of targeted foods to avoid wasting food and additional expense. Colin seemed less anxious around food, as he was not pressured to eat. He learned about food by labeling, counting, and describing.

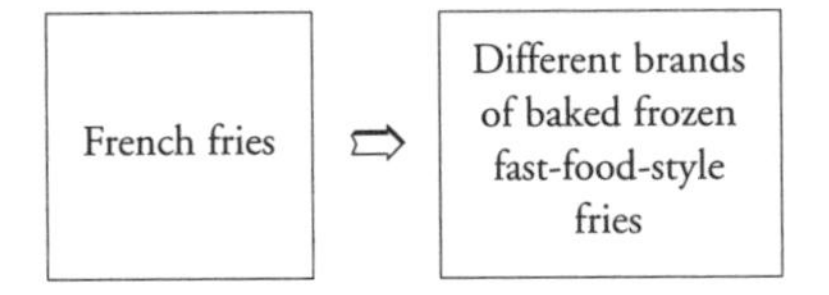

Masking Flavors: Colin was encouraged to dip his fries, and he started responding to new flavors, such as ranch dressing, honey mustard sauce, and ketchup. As we had hoped, once Colin felt comfortable with a variety of french fries, he was much more accepting of exposure to new food items. He explored new food with his hands and brought new foods to his mouth and started licking them. With repeated exposure Colin started accepting small bites of new foods. Ranch dressing and other sauces and condiments were used to introduce chicken nuggets and mask the flavor of the new food item until Colin could tolerate the taste without the masking flavor. This also opened the door to expanding Colin's tolerance of smooth foods. Now he is likely to tolerate strongly flavored smooth or pureed foods.

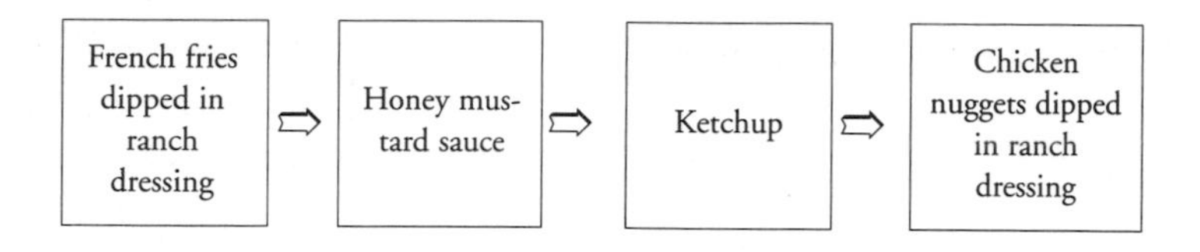

Novel Foods: Colin continued to like the aroma of sausage but could not tolerate the texture. But since he continued to show interest in spicy foods, we introduced novel spicy foods to his diet. Colin accepted chicken chipotle rolls and was soon eating them regularly. The team decided to go further and offered foods similar to the chipotle roll, such as pizza rolls, taquitos, and other snack rolls. Colin accepted all of these novel foods.

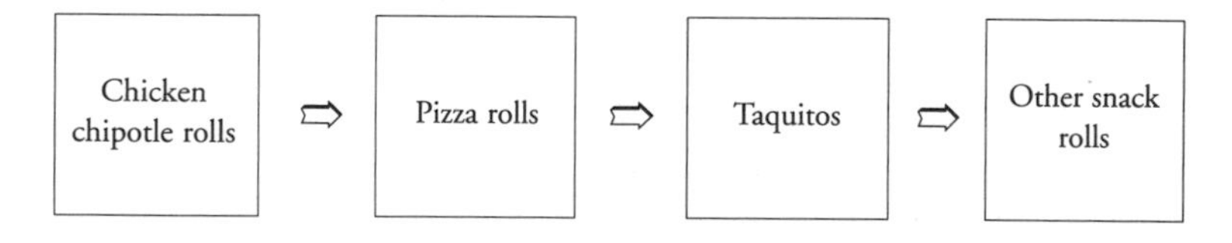

Liquids: Sherbet was added to Colin's carbonated beverages and eventually he accepted root beer floats. The team continued to modify ice cream to fruit-flavored milk shakes.

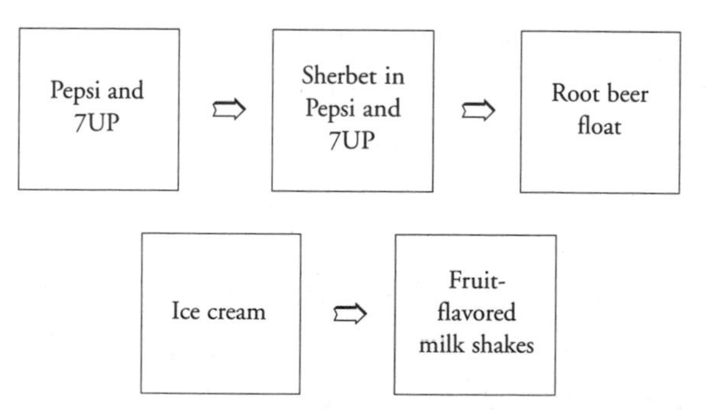

Progress Update The rating scales were used weekly to help the team and the family determine which foods should be offered first and how to continue to expand accepted foods, and to help establish long-term goal foods. Colin's weight gain and nutritional status improved.

FOOD CHAINING WITH CEREBRAL PALSY

Our feeding team treats many children with cerebral palsy (CP), but due to the nature of the condition, each food-chaining program is unique to the child. In other words, we cannot offer a typical food-chaining program example for cerebral palsy as we do for autism, vision impairment, and Down syndrome in this chapter. There are just too many variables. However, food chaining can help kids with CP, so if your child is having feeding problems, go to your pediatrician and begin the food-chaining process. Your pediatrician and a dietitian will be particularly important to your child's program, as kids with CP often have many medical and nutritional problems to contend with, such as weight gain and hydration issues, constipation, and aspiration.

DOWN SYNDROME

Down syndrome is a genetic condition in which an individual is born with forty-seven chromosomes instead of the usual forty-six and experiences delays in physical and intellectual development. It occurs in approximately one in every eight hundred live births, making it the most frequently occurring chromosomal disorder.

Most children with Down syndrome have mild to moderate impairments, and they are more like other children than they are different. While many kids with Down syndrome do require physical, speech, and developmental therapies, most attend their neighborhood schools, some in regular classes and others in special education classes. Some children have more significant needs and require a more specialized program.

Many children with Down syndrome have health complications beyond the usual childhood illnesses. Approximately 40 percent have congenital heart defects, and children with Down syndrome have a higher incidence of infection, respiratory, vision, and hearing problems as well as thyroid and other medical conditions. Many also struggle with feeding disorders, as they tend to have weak muscle tone and tire easily, which can affect their ability to eat. Many babies have trouble breast-feeding because their low muscle tone makes it hard for them to hold their tongue in place properly. Some babies with Down syndrome benefit from a special bottle system that helps them feed safely and successfully suck formula out of the bottle. Children with Down syndrome also tend to be slower to learn how to suck, swallow, and chew. They can be particularly sensitive to different textures and prefer smoother foods and familiar flavors. If your child has Down syndrome, a pediatric dietitian should monitor his weight and nutrition to make sure his weight doesn't get too high or too low.

BART'S FOOD-CHAINING PROGRAM

One-year-old Bart has Down syndrome and a heart condition

that required surgery at age six months. He has a long list of issues, including problems chewing and swallowing both food and liquid, frequent illness, constipation, and inadequate weight gain. He is a very picky eater who doesn't like to eat and never appears to be hungry. Bart received oral motor and feeding therapy prior to coming to the feeding team clinic, but he did not appear to progress in treatment. The local therapy team contacted our team for consultative care.

Family Goal: Bart's family wants to increase Bart's intake of food by mouth. Bart does not appear to enjoy eating, and his parents are afraid that tube feedings will decrease his desire to eat.

Step 1: Medical Evaluation Bart has Down syndrome and cardiac problems that required heart surgery at age six months. He has frequent colds and congestion. Bart has been the same weight for the past year, and his weight for age on the growth chart indicates failure to thrive. A g-tube had been placed when Bart was 10 months old. His family was given very little information on how to use the tube, and his feedings were not being adjusted by a medical professional at the time of our clinic visit. The amount of calories Bart was receiving through his g-tube and by mouth were not adequate for weight gain (his cardiac issues require him to have more calories than other children). The pediatrician's evaluation revealed that Bart has problems with constipation (constipation is more common in children with low muscle tone), which may also be decreasing his desire to eat. The pediatrician felt that Bart's constipation could be resolved with changes to his feedings. No other GI difficulties were diagnosed, and no further testing was ordered.

Step 2: Nutritional Evaluation The dietitian determined that Bart was not eating or drinking enough to gain weight. Bart was receiving only two tube feedings a day, which provided 12 ounces of PediaSure. His fluid intake was lower than it should have been, which might also have been contributing to his constipation. The dietitian recommended that Bart be fed five times a day, at 8:00 A.M., 11:00 A.M., 2:00 P.M., 5:00 P.M. and 8:00 P.M., and increased the amount of PediaSure he was getting to 30 ounces a day. The tube feedings would be given after he had eaten his pureed food by mouth. The amount of water Bart was receiving in his g-tube was adjusted to meet his needs and hopefully improve his constipation. In addition, the tube-feeding formula was changed to one that contained fiber. The nutritionist instructed Bart's parents not to offer him any food or liquid in between feedings. She showed Bart's family how to adjust his tube feedings if he had a good meal and consumed a larger quantity than normal by mouth. When Bart's nutritional status improved, he would likely eat more by mouth and his tube feedings could be decreased. First, his nutrition must be improved by using his tube more often to help him reach that goal.

Step 3: Feeding Evaluation The speech therapist's assessment revealed that Bart has weak muscles in his face. Bart's tongue regularly protrudes from his mouth. He has trouble closing his lips around a spoon and he is unable to chew food well. Bart is also unable to drink liquid well because he has not mastered the suck/swallow/breathe sequence (see chapter 4 for more information).

The speech therapist was concerned that Bart might be aspirating food or liquid into his lungs when he swallowed, which would explain his frequent colds and congestion. She ordered a modified barium swallow study (see chapter 3 for detailed information on this test), and the test results supported her concern. She recommended that Bart's liquids be thickened to a nectarlike consistency to give him more control over the liquid in his mouth before and during the swallow. Children with Down syndrome sometimes limit the amount of liquid they take in because it goes down the wrong tube when they swallow. The speech therapist hoped that the thicker liquid consistency would get Bart to drink more. An oral motor program was developed to strengthen the muscles of Bart's cheeks, lips, and tongue to improve his eating skills and prevent problems related to mouth breathing and possible **malocclusion** due to abnormal tongue position. The therapist changed the bottle and nipple Bart used to take liquids to encourage a more active, coordinated suck/swallow/breathe sequence and help strengthen the oral facial muscles. The therapist also provided oral motor toys, such as whistles, kazoos, and a harmonica made for children as part of the oral motor therapy program.

Since some foods are hard for Bart to chew, the speech therapist recommended that these foods be pureed or mashed for him. His mother was instructed to rest the spoon on his lower lip and let him suckle the food off the spoon. This helped to activate and strengthen his upper lip. Bart needed a little more time and this suckling action to move the pureed food back into his mouth for swallowing. Bart responded well to highly flavored purees and mashed foods. It was concluded that the majority of Bart's meal should be pureed, as his oral motor skills are not adequate for more challenging foods, but the therapist suggested that Bart's parents offer a few bites of solid foods at each meal to help him learn more advanced feeding skills.

Step 4: Sensory Evaluation Bart is underresponsive to sensory input and needs therapy to address this. The occupational therapist also found that Bart needs better support to his body during meals, with support under his feet to give him the stability he needs to chew more efficiently.

Step 5: Behavioral Evaluation Bart was evaluated by a psychologist through a developmental clinic prior to coming to our team. He had IQ testing and a detailed assessment. He has moderate mental retardation and learns best with multisensory teaching methods. (If testing like this has not been completed for your child, he will need a referral for full evaluation.)

Team Recommendations

Bart needs to learn about food just like any other child. We recommended that he be made part of food preparation and that his parents engage him in food-related activities at home. (See Teaching Kids with Autism about Food on page 264 for activity ideas. These ideas can also be used for children with a variety of diagnoses.) Learning about food will help expand Bart's speech and language skills as well as his acceptance of new foods. We recommended that picture schedules be used at meals so that Bart knows what to expect (washing hands, setting the table, serving the food, eating, and cleaning up). We suggested that his parents try using a token bite strip to reinforce Bart for good eating. The tokens should be bright, colorful, and textured to help maintain Bart's attention to eating.

Therapy Referrals

Bart was receiving physical, occupational, speech, and developmental therapies weekly through the Early Intervention program, but they were not focused on his feeding problems. We developed a treatment plan and implemented a communication system between all providers. We recommended that the therapists videotape their treatment sessions to share with the other therapists on the team or demonstrate with photos and therapy logs how to implement their feeding recommendations at meals. We explained that the therapists needed to agree to form one plan and not try to execute four separate therapy plans. We also stressed the importance of their using consistent language and a consistent approach to feeding for Bart.

Step 6: The Food Chains

Bart prefers foods that are smooth but will accept some lumpy foods. He likes sweet, tart, and strongly flavored foods.

BART'S CORE DIET

Bart's core diet consists of small bites of mashed potatoes, baby food cereal, baby food fruits and vegetables, Cool Whip, mashed baked beans, pudding, and gravy. Bart enjoys sips of juice and soda. He gags on milk.

BART'S FOOD CHAIN

Bart's parents were instructed to select two foods to modify initially at one meal each day and to gradually start modifying the other foods in Bart's core diet. It's very important to move slowly and not overwhelm him with change. The rating scales should be used to record Bart's reactions to new foods and report ratings to the team.

BART'S FOOD-CHAINING PROGRAM

The goal of the program is to improve his ability to chew more table foods and reduce the amount of fork mashing required. Carbonation in small amounts was added to liquids to work on his swallowing skills, but only during speech therapy sessions.

Accepted Foods and Suggested Modifications

Mashed potatoes

Level I

- Add seasoned salt, garlic, sour cream, or cheese sauce to whipped potatoes, whipped sweet potato casserole, whipped glazed carrots to continue the preference for sweet flavor.

Level II

- Offer fork-mashed sweet potatoes with marshmallow or crunchy brown sugar toppings and cheesy potato soup for soft vegetables in a mixed texture.

Gravy

- Try beef, pork, chicken, or sausage gravy. Also offer cream soups, cheese soup, stew (pureed), pureed chicken and noodles, broth soups thickened with potato flakes, and Alfredo sauce.

Baby food cereal

Level I

- Blenderize Quaker oatmeal flakes or instant flakes prior to cooking to achieve a texture similar to baby food cereal. Try flavored oatmeal and add applesauce or pureed peaches to oatmeal. Brown sugar, Cool Whip, or vanilla pudding can also be added to oatmeal.

Level II

- Gradually increase the texture and move toward tolerance of regular oatmeal. You can try Cream of Wheat, although some children do not tolerate the texture.

Pudding, graham crackers

- Offer puddings/graham cracker mixes: whipped cheesecakes, desserts with crushed graham cracker crusts, old-fashioned banana pudding with graham crackers or vanilla wafers, key lime pie, cream pies, graham cracker–crust or chocolate cookie–crust desserts.

Mashed baked beans

- Add BBQ sauces (look for flavors similar to the baked beans with your sauce) to beans. Offer seasoned chili beans and chili sauce. Black beans or kidney beans can be offered if well seasoned with sauces or thickened soups.

Baby food fruit and vegetables

- Puree fresh fruits and vegetables and work into baby foods until he tolerates all pureed.

Soda and juice

- Soda: offer root beer and cola with ice cream added to make floats. The carbonated cold liquids in small amounts help with trigger time of the swallow. This will also work toward a goal of tolerating milk shakes. Ice cream will eventually be reduced but not thinned beyond nectar consistency.
  Juice: offer Hawaiian Punch with orange sherbet added, lemonade with lime sherbet added, and yogurt smoothies. Work toward the goal of accepting milk.

Cool Whip

- Offer textured Cool Whip fluff-type desserts (e.g., cottage cheese, Cool Whip, strawberry Jell-O powder, pureed pineapple or mandarin oranges), Cool Whip with whipped pumpkin or cream pies, and add to pureed fruits.

Progress Report: The PediaSure with fiber and increase of water by g-tube did help ease Bart's constipation problems. Bart's weight gain improved. Liquids continued to be a challenge, but his intake increased. Initially Bart required 24 to 30 ounces of PediaSure with fiber in his g-tube daily for catch-up growth. After six months of therapy and food chaining, his tube feedings were reduced to 16 ounces daily. The team feels Bart will continue to need his g-tube to supplement his oral feedings or at least to provide his fluid needs. Bart went quickly through some of his food chains. He accepted baked beans and BBQ sauce easily, with ratings of 9 and 10. Lemon-flavored yogurt, sherbet, and Cool Whip desserts were also strong favorites. Bart's parents found it very easy to add pureed fruits and vegetables to the stronger-flavored foods Bart preferred. He was slower to accept potatoes, but he did like gravies and cream soups with potato flakes added. He accepted finely ground meats found in ravioli and other pastas. Bart now likes to eat, and meals are no longer a struggle.

CHILDREN WITH VISUAL IMPAIRMENT

Our eyes and our brains must work together in order for us to see. The cornea, iris, lens, and retina all work together in the eyes to focus on light and images. Then the eyes use special nerves to send what we see to our brains, so our brains can process and recognize what we're seeing. If our eyes work correctly, this process happens almost instantly.

For children with visual impairment, this process does not work properly. They are usually born with the condition, and the problem can affect one or both eyes. Some visually impaired children live in total darkness and are considered blind. Others can still see a little light or shadows, but they can't see anything clearly.

Every one of our senses plays a major role in our ability to eat, but vision gathers the most information for the brain. Unlike hearing, for example, which is a sequential sense that gathers one piece of information at a time, vision gathers all sorts of information nearby and at a distance simultaneously. Only vision can perceive shape, size, color, distance, and spatial location in one glance.

A baby's early development depends on vision, because all

body systems require visual feedback for practice and refinement. So vision impairment can have a profound effect on a child's feeding skills, and many visually impaired children struggle with feeding problems. These children do best with coordinated care between an occupational therapist, speech pathologist, vision impairment teacher, an early intervention service provider, and their family to develop a feeding program that meets their specific needs. (Working with a therapist who specializes in visual impairment is crucial to the success of a visually impaired child's treatment program. Therapy must start early for these children, ideally as soon as a vision problem is diagnosed.) There are so many ways to improve a visually impaired child's feeding situation. A feeding team can introduce color-contrast place mats, plates, utensils, and cups. They can provide sensory trays or place mats. A rope light can be used to outline the outside borders of the tray. The team can help facilitate a sense of control and independence for these kids at meals. They can also teach your child how to explore and learn about food with their other senses.

HOPE'S FOOD-CHAINING PROGRAM

Six-year-old Hope is visually impaired and has been diagnosed with dysphasia and constipation that affects her appetite and desire to eat. She is on a feeding tube and eats only three teaspoons of food orally at each meal.

Family Goal: Hope's family wants to increase the amount of food she can eat by mouth.

Step 1: Medical Evaluation Hope has been diagnosed with global developmental delays, cortical visual impairment, dysphasia, constipation, and multiple risk factors that could have an impact on her health. GER was also suspected, and Hope's pediatrician started her on reflux medications. Hope required a twice-daily dose of milk of magnesia to help with her constipation. The pediatrician ordered a modified barium swallow study to rule out aspiration.

Step 2: Nutritional Evaluation Hope has a g-tube in for supplemental feedings. She receives PediaSure through the tube five times each day, for a total of 27 ounces daily. Hope takes a vitamin called Poly-Vi-Sol that provides her with extra vitamins. She accepts only 50 to 60 calories per day by mouth. The dietitian instructed the family on how to prepare and puree foods to a consistency Hope can tolerate. The family was also given suggestions for storing and freezing pureed foods. Since the PediaSure Hope was receiving also provides her with vitamins and minerals, the dietitian recommended her vitamin supplement be adjusted so she didn't ingest an excess amount of vitamins and minerals.

Step 3: Feeding Evaluation Since Hope suffers from dysphagia (swallowing problems), a modified barium swallow study was completed and revealed that Hope is safest with purees and small amounts of thickened liquids. Hope is not able to chew foods well, and giving her solid foods puts her at risk for choking and aspiration. The majority of liquids should be given via her g-tube. The speech therapist focused on oral therapy and improving Hope's feeding skills before working to expand her diet. Food was modified to make it easier for her to eat. The family was instructed to puree foods they were having at meals and to add additional broths, condiments, and gravies as needed to make the food the correct consistency. They used the Magic Bullet, a small food processor that can puree almost any food, to do this at home, when dining out, and at school.

Step 4: Sensory Evaluation Hope likes foods that are flavorful. Her tongue works best to move the food around in her mouth when her food is strongly flavored. It would not be appropriate to give Hope baby food because she is over one year of age, and baby food has a bland flavor. Hope receives sensory information while eating in a different manner because of her visual impairment. We had her parents close their eyes and allow someone to try to feed them to experience meals as Hope does. Her parents were advised to slow down, not rush her, and to allow Hope the time she needs to experience the meal. Texture or bright contrasting colors were added to her spoon and plate. A textured place mat was used to cue Hope that it was time to eat and prepare her for the transition to the mealtime setting. We also recommended that Hope have a seating evaluation with an occupational therapist and a physical therapist so modifications to her wheelchair's headrest could be made. Proper head positioning is crucial so Hope can swallow well.

Step 5: Behavioral Evaluation Hope becomes distressed when others attempt to feed her. She needs to be aware of the spoon coming toward her mouth. A hand-over-hand technique will allow Hope to hold the spoon with guidance from the feeder as needed when she is eating. The feeders were instructed to talk about the food that they were offering and use a consistent verbal phrase (i.e., one, two, three, *bite*) to help Hope anticipate and prepare for the spoon being brought to her mouth. Hope also prefers to smell a bite of food before bringing it to her mouth, and we recommended that the feeder offer her a chance to do this with each bite. We also recommended that the feeder offer one food at a time and not alternate among different foods on Hope's plate.

Step 6: The Food-Chaining Program Hope already had a team of therapists she worked with locally, so we made the following suggestions to Hope's family and her therapists:

Food Suggestions Offer Hope pureed fruits and vegetables, spaghetti sauce, gravies, yogurt smoothies, pudding, Cool Whip desserts, whipped cheesecakes, mashed potatoes and gravy, whipped sweet potato, sausage gravy, scrambled egg, and green bean or vegetable casseroles. Her family was instructed to avoid casseroles with rice, as rice puts Hope at high risk for choking.

Condiments Use condiments to add calories to pureed foods and make them easier to swallow. Condiments also provide strong flavor and are sensory-alerting, which appeals to Hope. We recommended adding A1 steak sauce, BBQ sauce, salsa, chili sauce, ketchup, mayo, Dijon mustard, regular mustard, French onion chip dip, cheese sauce, ranch dressing, or "green goddess" dressing to foods. We advised her parents to puree any food they were having at home and to add condiments, gravies, broth, or water to get the food to the appropriate consistency.

Soups We suggested offering Hope beef- and chicken-broth-based soups (broth soups can be thickened with instant potato flakes), French onion soup, taco soup, and cream soups.

Meats We suggested Crock-Pot–prepared meats because they are very tender and easy to puree. (Always add additional water, broth, or gravies when you puree meats.)

Prepackaged Dinners We suggested offering Hope convenience foods such as microwaveable dinners (Salisbury steak, macaroni, spaghetti, or turkey and gravy) because they are easy to puree for a quick meal.

Progress Report Hope made good progress in treatment. Her caregivers and school and therapy teams all followed the same approach at every meal and snack. She continued to rely on her g-tube for most liquids and a large part of her nutritional intake, but she learned to eat and enjoy a wider variety of new foods. Hope's intake increased and she ate more foods when they were offered in pureed form. She now receives 23 ounces of PediaSure each day by g-tube, which is less than before. Due to Hope's health needs, removing her feeding tube was never an option. Hope is growing well, her nutritional status is improved, she is happier at meals, and she's able to eat the same foods her family eats with continued modification in texture.

IF YOUR CHILD IS UNDERNOURISHED

In order for your child to grow and develop properly, he must get an adequate amount of calories and nutrients. As you read in chapter 1, your child's nutritional status is determined by tracking her weight, height, and head circumference (through age three) at each pediatrician visit. If your child is receiving a sufficient amount of calories and nutrients and is growing well, she should follow her projected growth curve. Alternatively, if she's not receiving adequate nutrition for growth, she will deviate from her projected growth curve, which indicates she may be undernourished. If your child is deemed undernourished and is unable to take in enough nutrition orally, tube feedings will likely be required.

TUBE FEEDINGS

Tube feedings are used for a variety of reasons. Children who are extremely premature, have failure to thrive, dysphagia, aspiration, severe heart or lung disease, neurological impairment, genetic disorders, and structural anomalies such as cleft palate or tracheoesophageal fistula may require tube feeding to get the nutrition they need. The decision to use tube feedings is usually made by a group of health professionals, including the pediatrician, gastroenterologist, dietitian (see chapter 2 for an in-depth discussion on the role of a pediatric dietitian in your child's feeding program), and other pediatric subspecialists.

Type of Tubes There are two types of tubes that are typically used for tube feedings: nasogastric and gastrostomy. Usually your team of doctors will recommend a particular tube for your child based on how long they expect she will need tube feedings as well as patient-related factors (such as how likely it is that the nasogastric tube will be pulled out accidentally or purposefully by the child) or parental concerns (such as the stress or difficulty you may encounter keeping a nasogastric tube in place). Nasogastric tubes, which are inserted through the nose and into the stomach, are often used for short periods of time (less than a few months). Gastrostomy tubes, which are surgically inserted directly into the stomach, are used for long-term feedings. Neither of these tubes is permanent, so when your child is able to maintain her nutritional and hydration status and take her medications by mouth, the tube can be removed.

Types of Feedings Once your child's tube is placed, it is time to determine how to administer the feedings. Feedings can be provided either by bolus or continuous drip. Bolus feedings are delivered several times a day (usually four to eight) and last from 10 to 30 minutes, depending on your child's tolerance for them. They require less equipment than continuous feedings, are often less expensive, and are more convenient for you to administer. They also allow your child more mobility and normality in everyday activities because she is not connected to a pump. However, some children cannot tolerate bolus feedings and may experience gagging and retching, nausea, vomiting, or abdominal pain. These children may require either continuous feedings or a combination of smaller bolus feedings and continuous feedings.

Continuous feedings are provided by a feeding pump. The formula is put in a feeding bag that has tubing that connects to your child's feeding tube. A pump administers the feedings over a several-hour period. Usually children receive these feedings for 8 to 12 hours at night while they sleep.

It's important to note that not all children will use a feeding tube in the same way. In order for a tube feeding to work, it must be compatible with your child's tolerance for it, your family situation, and your child's medical condition. Some children only need to use their tube for hydration and are able to get the rest of their nutrition by mouth. Other children are unable to meet their nutritional needs by mouth and need the tube to help them grow and get extra calories.

Transitioning to Oral Feedings Transitioning your child from tube feedings to oral feedings is a complex process and it should be directed by your child's ability and her tolerance for oral feedings. The transition process should be both achievable and pleasurable for your child, and it should not in any way compromise her health or growth. There are several criteria your child must meet before she is ready to transition to oral feedings.

First and foremost, if your child suffers from a medical condition that required her to start tube feedings, the medical condition must be resolved before she can transition to table foods. For example, if your child had a tube placed because she was aspirating food into her lungs, her doctor will need to perform a repeat modified barium swallow study (see chapter 3 for a description of this study) to make sure it is safe for your child to begin oral feedings.

Your child should also be well nourished, have grown appropriately as a result of the tube feedings, and be in overall good health. For example, if your child has a seizure disorder and is currently having problems that require her medications to be adjusted, this is not a time to transition her to oral feedings.

Your child's health-care team must also take into account what type of feeding your child is receiving as they consider how and when to transition her. A child who receives continuous drip feeds will not have the same hunger and satiety cues as a child who receives bolus feeds, since bolus feeds more closely mimic meal- and snack-time intervals. Many children on continuous drip feedings are first transitioned to a bolus-feeding regimen before moving to oral feedings. That said, it's certainly not impossible to transition a child who receives continuous drip feedings directly to oral feedings. Hunger is our friend and often helps with the transition.

Another key factor is that your child must demonstrate interest in eating orally and find doing so pleasurable. Your child's health-care team will pay close attention to her interactions with food. If she exhibits negativity toward table foods, or gags or vomits, this is probably not the right time to transition her. Her doctors will need to get your child more comfortable with food first before making the jump to oral feedings.

Once your child is ready to make the transition, there are several ways her feedings can be adjusted to accomplish this goal. Your child's health-care team may reduce the calories provided by the tube feedings by 25 percent to see if your child is able to make up the difference on her own. They may have your child skip a tube feeding to see if it will make her more interested in eating a meal. Some children even forgo tube feedings for a day or two (under close supervision) so their health-care team can see if they are able to meet their needs by mouth. Your child's response to this initial "trial" will help her health-care team determine how best to approach the weaning of tube feedings.

A good health-care team will let your child set the pace. They will listen to what her words and body language are telling them and customize her weaning to make the transition both pleasurable and successful. For instance, if your child exhibits signs that they have cut back too much on calories and have put too much pressure on her to eat (making mealtimes negative for her), her health-care team will adjust her weaning accordingly. They will do the same if it appears that they have not cut back enough and your child is still not interested in eating. Your child's weight will be monitored closely throughout the process. Usually the feeding tube will not be removed until your child is able to take liquids and solids by mouth and maintain growth for a period of at least six months.

ANDY'S STORY

Andy came to see our team at age 18 months. Born one month premature, he had pulmonary hypertension during his neonatal stay in the hospital, which required ventilation. He was also diagnosed with delayed gastric emptying, reflux, oral aversion, and failure to thrive.

As an infant, Andy always had problems eating. "It was very difficult to get him to take a bottle. We had to distract him during feedings to get him to eat," says his mother, Joanne. "At three months of age, we switched him from a cow's-milk formula to a soy formula to see if this would help with feedings. When that didn't work, his pediatrician changed him to a hypoallergenic formula, which he was on until age eight months. I started him on baby foods at seven months of age but stopped because the pediatrician was concerned about his growth."

At one year, Andy was started on table foods, but again, with little success. He continued to fail to thrive, disliked eating, and would gag when sitting in his high chair, both at the anticipation and at the sight of food. By 17 months of age, doctors put Andy on bolus tube feedings, but still he gained very little weight and began vomiting. Initially Andy was offered meals orally and then bolus feedings of a pediatric supplement five times each day. When that didn't work, the tube feedings were changed to smaller boluses, and continuous nighttime drip feedings were added. Andy continued to vomit and continued to gag and refuse his oral feedings. This is the point at which Andy's parents brought him to us for help.

During our initial appointment, we decided that the bolus feedings were not working for Andy. In fact, they were making him more aversive to his oral feedings during the day. We put him on a continuous nighttime drip feeding. We also showed his parents how to handle Andy's mealtime behaviors such as gagging and vomiting (see chapter 5 for an in-depth discussion on the behavior modification portion of the food-chaining program).

After about a month, Andy stopped vomiting, and his parents were able to begin some oral feedings again. Andy gained weight very well on this feeding regimen and continued to make gains when his parents started to offer food twice a day. At this point he also began to work with a speech therapist. His parents found that they were offering the same foods over and over again because they knew Andy would eat them, so we discussed expanding his food repertoire using the food-chaining program.

At this point Andy started drinking a high-calorie shake that his mom had created. We began weaning Andy's tube feedings at night, and his food intake gradually increased without significant decreases in nighttime feedings. When his tube feedings were stopped at 22 months of age, initially Andy had a slight weight loss. His weight stayed the same for two months before he was started on a medication to help stimulate his appetite. Then his weight began to increase again, and he was weaned from this medication. He grew steadily until 30 months of age, at which point the gastrostomy tube was removed. Today he continues to grow appropriately and eat a normal toddler diet. If we had continued Andy on the bolus feedings, the transition to oral feedings would probably have taken longer because the vomiting had made eating a negative experience for him. Andy's story is a good example of how a child really must direct his own feeding program and transition.

A FINAL WORD

In this chapter, we have offered several examples of how we modify meals and develop programs for children with special needs. It's important to understand that there is no "one way" to do therapy with a child with special needs. For instance, not every autistic child will benefit from a treatment plan like the ones we describe above. Every child is different and needs his or her own unique treatment program to be successful. Many times family support, respite services, and education regarding rights, laws, trust funds, and care later in life need to be part of the treatment program. We are aware that feeding is only the tip of the iceberg when it comes to the challenges you and your family may be facing. What we've tried to do is give you practical ideas that may improve meals for you and your family. Any child with special needs requires careful medical evaluation before starting a program, and nutrition should be the number one priority in treatment.

Appendix 1

Sample Food Chains

Following are sample food-chaining programs for an infant, a young child, and a teenager. These are real food-chaining programs, created for children who have been treated by our feeding team. The names have been changed to protect their privacy.

Keisha's Food Chain

Eleven-and-a-half-month-old Keisha's parents brought her to see us because she is gagging on stage II foods and solids (Cheerios) to the point of vomiting. She cries at meals and is having difficulty transitioning to a sippy cup.

Step 1: Medical Evaluation Keisha's overall medical evaluation was unremarkable, but her GI evaluation revealed that she has a history of frequent spitting up. She spit up often but there did not appear to be a pattern of reflux. Her parents reported that she would spit up five minutes after feeding or up to two hours after feeding. She had no history of blue spells or breathing problems related to reflux. She gained weight well and never demonstrated any kind of aversion to bottle- or spoon-feeding until she moved from stage I foods to stage II foods and the texture changed.

Step 2: Nutrition Evaluation Keisha demonstrated good weight gain. She accepted a variety of stage II baby food fruits and vegetables, but was starting to show a more negative response to baby food meats. Keisha took a good volume of liquid by bottle but was having trouble transitioning to cup feeding. The dietitian recommended that Keisha's parents not push cup drinking for all liquid intake until Keisha was ready. She was also old enough to start tastes of puddings, yogurts, and gravies.

Step 3: Feeding Evaluation Keisha demonstrated good coordination of the suck/swallow/breathe sequence. However, she had a weak lip seal on the bottle nipple and appeared to be taking in a large amount of air while feeding. The speech therapist switched Keisha to a Dr. Brown's bottle and replaced the nipple with the Parents' Choice nipple. The bottle is designed to reduce air intake while feeding, and the replacement nipple is slightly wider, providing better lip seal. The therapist planned to eventually move back to the narrower Dr. Brown's nipple as she continued to work on improving Keisha's lip seal. Her pacifier was replaced with a Soothie brand pacifier to also work on lip seal. This pacifier is slightly longer and makes contact farther back on her tongue. This would provide more contact to her tongue and help desensitize her strong gag reflex. Keisha seemed to be sensitive to the hard spout of the cup, and because of her weak lip seal, she could not control liquid well in her mouth.

The therapist selected the Nuby soft-spout cup for her, and the silicone spout helped Keisha successfully drink small amounts of liquids from the cup. Keisha would continue to take liquids from her bottle and her cup until her cup drinking skills improve. Keisha also appeared to be sensitive to the mixed lumpy texture of stage III baby foods. The therapist suggested that the family puree table foods to a smooth consistency and allow Keisha time to get used to the stronger flavor of the puree. She recommended that the Nuk brush, a textured teether, be used as a spoon. Keisha enjoyed biting on the brush dipped in her purees. This encouraged development of chewing and biting patterns but required Keisha to swallow only a pureed consistency. Gagging can be very frightening to a child and can create a strong aversive response to eating. The team felt that mixed textures were going to be the most challenging for Keisha.

Step 4: Sensory Evaluation Keisha does not appear to have significant sensory issues even though she has a strong gag reflex. The occupational therapist modified her seating at meals. A First Years booster seat was recommended. A variety of teether toys was offered to help desensitize her gag reflex further. The Nuk brush and a textured spoon were used at meals, and the occupational therapist provided suggestions to help Keisha develop her independent feeding skills.

Step 5: Behavioral Evaluation Keisha is a very inquisitive child, and her developmental skills are on track. She quickly picked up on her parents' anxiety at meals. When Keisha gagged, her mother was afraid she would vomit, so she grabbed a towel and put it under her chin during gagging spells. Keisha became alarmed and cried when this occurred. The team explained that placing the towel under her chin might actually have the negative effect of encouraging Keisha to vomit. A behavioral vomiting pattern could develop. Keisha's family provided videotapes of meals at home for analysis by the team. The behavioral psychologist viewed the tapes with the family and identified reactions that might result in further feeding issues. Her parents were instructed to show no reaction when gagging occurred and to comfort Keisha with a soft voice and touch. The therapist explained that gagging was a normal part of learning to eat, and gave Keisha's family food ideas designed to reduce her risk of gagging.

Step 6: The Food Chain Keisha was transitioned from baby food to pureed table food. Fruits and vegetables were targeted first. Keisha's parents would rate her reactions to foods and the feeding specialist would provide specific foods based on ratings. Flavor would be changed before texture.

Accepted Foods and Suggested Modifications

Stage II baby foods fruits and vegetables

Goal: Pureed fruits and vegetables

- Puree small amounts of real fruits and vegetables. Work in a small amount of this puree to the stage II baby food. You may need to start with as little as ½ tsp.
- Initial goal will be to get Keisha to all pureed fruits/vegetables with seasoning added as tolerated.

Tip: Pureed food can be stored and frozen in ice cube trays. Trays should then be wrapped in plastic and placed inside a large Ziploc bag. Place a paper towel inside the bag to absorb moisture.

New food ideas:

Tiny amounts of new foods will be offered as tolerated on the Nuk brush, pacifier, or textured spoon. (We are introducing new foods because Keisha may be gagging on the bland flavor of baby food and may not gag on more flavorful food that provides more sensory feedback.)

- Thinned mashed potatoes and gravy. Some children only tolerate gravies without the potatoes. Try offering chicken, beef, pork, or sausage gravies to expose to flavor in a texture she can tolerate.
- Cream soups
- Thickened broths or broth-based soups thickened with instant potato flakes (French onion, vegetable, tortilla soup, chicken or beef broth soups)
- Baby yogurt
- Puddings
- Tastes of spaghetti sauce

Stage II baby food meats

(toward which she is showing more aversion)

- Small amounts of gravy or thickened broth may be added to baby food meats to make them more palatable and head off gagging.
- When modified baby foods are accepted well, continue to advance diet.
- Puree/process meats such as spaghetti sauce, Salisbury steak, meat loaf, seasoned taco meat, hamburger, Crock-Pot–cooked chicken, and add gravy, cream soups.
- Another idea is to offer small amounts of pureed or ground meat with mashed potatoes and gravy. (If Keisha is gagging, the mashed potatoes may be too thick.)

New food ideas

- Any broth soup can be thickened with instant potato flakes. Some children respond well to tortilla soup,

French onion soup, and other strong flavors. Think of all the possibilities and flavors of soup.

- Tomato soup or cream soups may be tolerated (cheese, potato, stews). You can also puree vegetables and add to these soups and mixtures.
- Uniform textured foods (foods that have lumps that are all the same size and the texture is lumpy throughout the food) can be offered. Try cottage cheese or cottage cheese in a dessert made with Cool Whip/Jell-O powder and tapioca pudding. These foods are more likely to be tolerated than a smooth food with lumps.
- Whipped yogurts may be accepted.
- Any smooth food can be made a uniform texture by crushing a crunchy topping and working it in to the puree. You can crush any of the following foods: Durkee onions, Funyuns, potato chips, saltine or club crackers, graham crackers, shortbread cookies, chocolate cookies (Oreos), pretzels, tostada chips, Rice or Corn Chex, cereals or oatmeal/brown sugar crunchy toppings. Stir these foods into the puree to achieve a uniform texture.
- Some children also like granola and Grape-Nuts Flakes added to their smooth foods; however, these foods may pose a choking risk for some children.
- Gradually transition to offering these foods as finger foods (not the pretzels) as directed by your therapist.

New food ideas to be offered when Keisha is demonstrating adequate oral motor skills for these foods.

- Offer pancakes, small bites of a frozen waffle and French toast, muffins, fruit breads, biscuits, toast, cheese quesadilla, fruit bars, and plain Pop-Tarts. (Some children do better with foods in this category instead of foods of mixed consistency.)

Chloe's Food-Chaining Program

Four-year-old Chloe was brought to see our team because she was eating very few foods. She refused to try most new foods, and the ones she did try made her gag. She also appeared to have an extreme sensitivity to the aroma of foods.

Family Goal: Chloe's family wants her to start eating pasta, breads, meat, and vegetables.

Step 1: Medical Evaluation Chloe is in good health. Her medical and developmental histories are unremarkable.

Step 2: Nutrition Evaluation Chloe eats six foods and one liquid. She will not accept any fruit, vegetables, or meat. She takes her lunch to school. Her mother reported that one day she forgot her lunch and refused to try anything on her hot lunch tray. She pushed the tray away immediately. Chloe eats approximately a third of her lunch at school and then finishes it in the car during the drive home. When she arrives home from school she also wants to eat and then she eats very poorly at dinner. The dietitian suggested that Chloe have a small snack in the car, but no other food until dinner. This gentle appetite manipulation may significantly improve her intake at the evening meal.

Step 3: Feeding Evaluation Chloe has a significantly restricted food repertoire. She will only eat pepperoni, yogurt, pretzels, crackers, fruit roll-ups, and Kraft macaroni and cheese, and she drinks only chocolate milk. The foods Chloe accepts are of a uniform texture—they do not change during chewing. Her parents are instructed to offer new foods with the understanding that she will need time to learn about the food before eating it. She will need to see the food, smell it, and touch it with utensils, and then with her hands. Her parents should offer a new food at one snack time or one mealtime each day at first and then gradually expand to more food items. Chloe can help pick a new food she wants to try at a meal. Shopping together or watching cooking shows will also teach her about food.

Step 4: Sensory Evaluation Chloe had a sensory processing assessment with the occupational therapist, and testing revealed sensitivity to smells of food, but no true sensory processing disorder. The family will keep track of the aromas of food and other smells at home to share with the team. Lunchtime at school may be more difficult for Chloe due to the variety of aromas from the cafeteria. Chloe can participate in cooking to help desensitize her to these smells. If she cannot do that yet, she can be in a room close to the kitchen until she can tolerate being in the room while food is prepared. Chloe can also help set the table or participate in other mealtime preparations to expose her to the aromas of food.

Step 5: Behavioral Evaluation The team developed a feeding book about Chloe for her mother to read to her at home. The feeding book will help Chloe learn why it is important for her health and appearance to eat well. Chloe successfully tried one new food and liked caramel apples. She should be praised for her willingness to try new foods. Chloe still indicates that she does not wish to expand her diet. The team suggested that Chloe's parents set up a reward system where she gets stickers for progress made that earns her a special treat at the end of each week. The team noted that Chloe receives a great deal of attention for her picky eating and that this may be causing the problem to persist. Her parents should offer her meals and snacks on a schedule and stay within the time limit. If Chloe chooses not to eat, she will have to live with the consequence of that choice, which is hunger.

Therapy Referral: Chloe will be scheduled to see the behavioral psychologist to help her family develop a consistent method of handling her food refusals and other behavioral concerns.

Step 6: The Food Chain

Accepted Foods and Possible Modifications

Macaroni and cheese

- Chloe likes Kraft macaroni and cheese. At first a modification may be that you cut the pieces of macaroni into smaller pieces to show her that even though it looks a little different, it is still the same.
- **Next change:** You can use the Kraft macaroni and cheese powder, milk, and butter and add it to pasta noodles of different shapes and sizes (shells, elbow macaroni, rotini, etc.). This will maintain taste but give a different noodle shape and texture. This is a good cooking activity to share with Chloe.
- When she tolerates the changes above, try the type of new pasta that she likes best and make macaroni and cheese with Velveeta cheese. Some parents add a little of the Kraft powder for color and flavor. See if she can get used to a variation in macaroni and cheese. This is another good cooking activity for Chloe.

- Later in treatment, pasta can be used with other sauces (Alfredo, marinara, chili mac, buttered). Chloe can put tiny tastes of these new sauces on her pasta with a paintbrush, or she can dip the pasta noodle in the sauce.

Chicken nuggets

- Try McDonald's chicken nuggets. You may want to try Chicken Selects.
- Offer other chicken nuggets, too, such as Sonic popcorn chicken, Burger King chicken fries, and KFC popcorn chicken.
- Try Tyson or other brands of chicken strips at home (baked on a baking stone is the best health option).
- When Chloe accepts these, consider trying pieces of fried chicken and eventually a fried chicken leg.
- Next levels: Baked chicken with a crunchy topping (Bisquick, Shake 'n Bake, etc.).
- New food ideas based on chicken: fried fish (Long John Silver's or McDonald's fish fillet, popcorn shrimp, fried scallops). Also try breaded pork tenderloin, breaded vegetables/cheese sticks. (Cheddar cheese may be easier, as mozzarella can be too stringy and can cause choking.)
- Eventually move to baked chicken dipped in a sauce such as BBQ or honey mustard or ranch dressing. Some children love hot wings and teriyaki chicken.
- Turkey and other fowl can be introduced.
- As Chloe tolerates baked chicken, other meats may be offered. Small bites of deli meats or other meats may be tolerated, such as thin-sliced roast beef, ham, salami, and pastrami.

Fruit

- Fruit can be added to milk shakes or yogurt smoothies, or dipped in chocolate or cream cheese dips.
- Fruit can be topped with nuts or whipped cream.
- Fruit pies or crisps/pastries may be accepted.
- Offer fruit chips.
- Fruit jellies/preserves can be added to a variety of breads, mini bagels, rolls, or croissants to introduce a variety of bread products.
- Try fruit and peanut butter.
- Offer Chloe fruit roll-ups.

Chocolate milk

- Offer chocolate milk with ¼ to ½ packet of Carnation Instant Breakfast added. Increase amount of Carnation Instant Breakfast as tolerated. This is a good way to get minerals and vitamins, and it tastes very pleasant. (Vanilla Carnation Instant Breakfast is fine to add, as the chocolate has a bit of an aftertaste.)
- Try different varieties of chocolate milk.
- Offer hot chocolate with whipped cream, chocolate sprinkles, or marshmallows.
- Try milk shakes (whipped cream and a cherry can be added). Some children also like decorative straws to make snacks fun.
- Move from chocolate pudding to chocolate pie. If pie crust is accepted, you can offer a variety of cream pies and fruit-and-cream pies.

The pie crust may also be chained to the crust of a chicken pot pie or quiche.

Novel foods

- Don't be afraid to offer small portions of a new food at each meal (1 to 2 Tbsp). You just want her to tolerate it on her plate. No pressure to eat it.

Rachel's Food-Chaining Program

Fifteen-year-old Rachel is active and involved in sports. However, she has been a picky eater since age one, and her entire family is feeling increasing stress at meals. Rachel's food selectivity is now affecting her social life.

Team Assessment

Rachel does not have any underlying medical issues or oral motor/swallowing problems, but her nutritional status is an area of concern. Rachel's problems with food started with the transition from baby food to solids. She started avoiding certain types of food, primarily meats, vegetables, and dairy products. She preferred waffles and rice, and for a while she ate most fruits, but then those too dropped out of her diet. Nothing has changed in her diet preferences since her toddler years. Now Rachel is a growing teenager and an athlete. She is weight-appropriate but malnourished. Her hair is falling out. Rachel will accept milk shakes, and that gives us a quick way to improve her nutritional status. The team talked at length with Rachel and her family about her issues with food. Her visit with the psychologist revealed that she did not show signs of an eating disorder, such as anorexia or bulimia. Talking about how her sensitivities with food were affecting and limiting her choices in life motivated Rachel to make changes, but she felt frustrated by her family's pushing her to eat.

Rachel's feeding issues appear to be sensory based. She likes foods that are all one texture, even during the act of chewing, such as rice and pasta. She will sometimes eat watermelon and strawberries, but not often. Rachel does not put sauces on her pasta and she likes Kraft macaroni and cheese, which is flavorful but remains one texture. She will eat pizza, but the sauce must be smooth, with no chunks. Again, she is looking for no texture changes, no surprises. When we explained Rachel's sensory profile to her, she had a much better understanding of her struggle with food. Her family was also relieved when they learned that we could help develop a program to improve her tolerance of a wider variety of foods.

Core Diet Rachel's core diet consists of waffles, rice, macaroni and cheese, rotini noodles, potato chips, mashed potatoes, bagel bites, chicken nuggets, french fries, nacho chips, cheese pizza, candy, and protein bars.

Modifications: Rachel's core diet consists mainly of snack foods, but there is still great potential to expand her diet.

Rice

Since she accepts rice, Rachel may also accept fried rice and long-grain rice, which would allow us to introduce Chinese dishes. Rachel is close to dating age and may be motivated to learn to eat out at restaurants. But we must be careful not to overwhelm her. She should work a thickened broth into the rice at first so she won't be overwhelmed by the mixed texture. She may also eventually like rice pudding or tapioca pudding. Other flavors of pudding can be explored in desserts or through cream pies.

Kraft Macaroni and Cheese

Rachel has a preference for pasta and cheesy flavor. We may be able to build on those preferences to introduce new foods. Pastas can be modified with butter or shredded mozzarella cheese. A small amount of marinara or Alfredo sauce can be stirred into her pasta to see if she likes it.

Potato Chips

There are many flavors of chips and we can expose her to these new tastes and help her experience flavors like sour cream and onion that might eventually be modified to become a baked potato with sour cream. There is a link between these two foods. Also try potato chips in cheddar, salt and vinegar, and BBQ flavors. Dips and ranch dressing should be offered for dipping potato chips. Preferred snack products such as Doritos, Funyuns, and cheese puffs will be used to teach Rachel about the flavors she prefers and how to find those features in other foods. Rachel is in a rut; she is eating the same thing all the time. Modifying her snack foods will give her a variety of sensory experiences but not overwhelm her. Vegetables will also be targeted using vegetable chips. Chips made from sweet potatoes and beets are very crunchy and taste great.

Pizza, Pasta, and Chicken Nuggets

Pizza is a food that is important to social life. Rachel is motivated to improve her tolerance for a variety of brands of pizza so she can have more social interaction with her friends. Different types of pizza can be offered—thin crust, thick crust, pizza rolls, pizza bread, and calzones. Zucchini, tomato, or squash can be pureed and added in small amounts to her pizza sauce. Start at ½ teaspoon at first and increase from there. Later in her treatment, toppings can be added to her pizza to further expand her diet. Since Rachel likes chicken nuggets, pasta, and pizza sauce, the team targeted chicken Parmesan as a goal meal for restaurants (Rachel was told that she could order the sauce on the side). This allowed her to go out socially with her family and have a meal. She could also order this meal when she started dating. The team designed food chains to expand breaded meats, pastas, and sauces such as Alfredo sauce.

Candy/Fruit

Rachel likes candy and used to like all fruits, but they have dropped out of her diet. At one time fruit worked for her, so we will try to bring it back by masking the flavor of the fruit with chocolate sauce. We will prepare a fruit and chocolate fondue or offer chocolate-dipped strawberries or other dipped fruits. The amount of chocolate will be gradually phased out to help Rachel experience the true flavor of the fruit. Rachel may also like cream cheese–based fruit dips to combine her sweet tooth with fresh fruit. Another easy solution for Rachel is adding Carnation Instant Breakfast mix and fresh fruits to her milk shakes.

Novel Foods

Rachel was motivated to learn to eat new foods so she could go to fast-food restaurants and feel more comfortable at lunch with her friends. Rachel agreed to try salad with ranch dressing. She felt that this was a food that did not change excessively by chewing, and she understood from her sensory profile that she might be successful eating it.

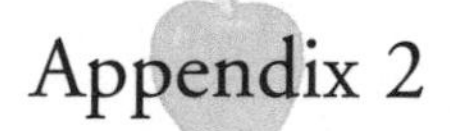

Appendix 2

Feeding Your Baby and Young Child

Feeding Your Baby

Age birth to two years

Please note that these are general guidelines. Every baby is different and will progress at his own rate. Your baby may eat more or less than this guide suggests.

AGE	FOOD GROUP	FOODS	DAILY SERVINGS	SUGGESTED SERVING SIZE
0–4 Months	Milk	Breast milk or iron-fortified infant formula	8–12 or on demand	
		0–1 mos		2–4 oz.
		1–2 mos	6–8	3–6 oz.
		2–3 mos	5–7	4–7 oz.
		3–4 mos	4–7	6–8 oz.
			4–6	
4–6 Months	Milk	Breast milk or formula	4–6 4–6	6–8 oz.
	Grain	Baby cereal with iron	2	1–2 Tbsp.
6–9 Months	Milk	Breast milk or formula	3–5 3–5	6–8 oz.
	Grain	Baby cereal with iron	2	2–4 Tbsp.
		Bread, crackers	Offer	½ slice, 2 crackers
	Fruit	Fruit	2	
		Baby fruit juice	Offer	2–3 Tbsp.
	Vegetables	Vegetables	2	2 ounces (from cup)
	Meats	Chicken, beef, pork	2	2–3 Tbsp.
				1–2 Tbsp.

FEEDING TIPS
• Nurse your baby at least 5–10 minutes on each breast. Your milk supply will increase as your baby needs and demands more milk. • Breast-fed infants may need to nurse one or more times during the night. • Six to eight wet diapers a day is a good sign. • Hold your baby upright when feeding. • Do not prop a bottle. • Do not add cereal to a bottle unless recommended by your doctor. This does not make babies sleep longer. • Do not force your baby to finish a bottle. A baby will turn their head away, push the nipple out of his mouth, or fall asleep when he is finished.
• Your baby is ready for solids when he: 1. can hold head up steadily and sit with support 2. does not push the spoon out of his mouth with his tongue 3. can turn his head to stop a feeding 4. opens his mouth when he sees food • Begin with rice cereal and feed him only one new cereal per week. Do not use an "infant feeder." • Do not add salt or sugar to the cereal. • It's ok to offer up to 2 ounces water per day in a cup
• Use a baby-size spoon. • Do not force your baby to eat a food. • Meals times will be messy. Be patient. • Minimize distractions during feeding time. • Take the amount from the jar for one feeding. Refrigerate the remaining food. • Feed only one new fruit or vegetables every 3–4 days. • Try giving water or fruit juice in a cup. Do not use juice as a substitute for breast milk or formula. Do not offer orange, grapefruit, or pineapple juice until 12 months of age. • Add strained fruits and vegetables. Add mashed or finely chopped fruits and cooked vegetables later on. • Add strained meats. Feed only one new meat every 3–4 days. • Feed your baby in a high chair and try to feed him at the same time as the rest of the family. • Around 8 months, offer small pieces of well cooked vegetables, soft fruits, or crackers. This will encourage self-feeding skills. • Never leave baby alone while eating. Babies can choke easily and need supervision. **• Wait until your baby's first birthday to give milk, honey, strawberries, citrus fruits, chocolate, fish, and peanut butter. If your family has a high risk for food allergies, avoiding shellfish and peanuts until age 3 is recommended.**

AGE	FOOD GROUP	FOODS	DAILY SERVINGS	SUGGESTED SERVING SIZE
9–12 Months	Milk	Breast milk or formula Cheese Plain yogurt Cottage cheese	3–4 3–4 Offer	6–8 oz. ½ oz. ¼ cup ¼ cup
	Grain	Baby cereal with iron Bread, crackers, dry oat cereal rings, Soft cooked noodles	2–3	2–4 Tbsp. 2 crackers Offer
	Fruit	Fruit Baby fruit juice	2	2–4 Tbsp. 3 oz. (from cup)
	Vegetables	Vegetables	2–3	2–4 Tbsp.
	Meats/Meat Substitutes	Chicken, turkey, beef, pork, cooked, dried beans or egg yolks	2	2–4 Tbsp.
12–24 Months	Milk	Whole milk, yogurt cheese, cottage cheese	4	½ cup ½ oz. ¼ cup
	Grain	Cereal, pasta, rice bread, muffins, rolls crackers	6	¼ cup ½ 2 crackers
	Fruit	Cooked, juice whole	2–3	¼ cup ½ medium
	Vegetable	Cooked, juice whole	2–3	¼ cup ½ medium
	Meat/ Meat Substitutes	Fish, chicken, turkey, beef, pork, cooked dried beans, egg	2	1 oz. ¼ cup 1 egg

FEEDING TIPS
• Give your baby a baby-size spoon and let him try to feed himself. • Be patient. Babies make a mess when they feed themselves. • Offer finger foods with more texture to promote self feeding. Use mostly soft table foods. • Wait until your baby's first birthday to feed him egg whites. Some babies are sensitive to the egg whites. It's okay to give him the yolks. • Offer a cup at every meal. **• Offer the following foods only when your baby has a full set of teeth because they may cause choking: apple chunks or slices, grapes, hot dogs, sausages, peanut butter, popcorn, nuts, seeds, round candies, and hard chunks of uncooked vegetables.**
• Your toddler should be weaned from baby foods. • Add whole milk now. • Encourage your toddler to drink from a cup rather than a bottle. • Toddlers may not eat as much as they did the first year of life because growth slows down. • Offer small portions and never force your toddler to eat. • Respect your toddler's likes and dislikes. Offer rejected foods over and over again. • Feed your toddler the same foods as the rest of the family. • Set a good example. Your toddler will tend to like to eat the same foods you like. • Offer at least 2–3 snacks every day.

Feeding Your Child

Ages two to six years

Growth, Independence, Appetite

Children do not grow as quickly during this time. Their activity level will affect their appetite, and it's normal for children to eat only one good meal a day. This is also the age when children begin to want to do more things on their own. This desire for independence can take a toll on eating, and many children refuse to eat a particular food or to eat at all.

Encouraging Variety

You should offer your child food choices from at least three food groups during a meal, and offer different types of foods throughout the day.

The best way to encourage your child to eat different types of food is to eat them yourself. When you offer your child a new food, do so in a nonpressuring way and allow your child to decide whether to eat the new food. Talk about the food and teach your child how it will taste, feel, and smell. If he won't try it, don't give up—offer it again at another meal. It's common for children to reject a food 12 to 15 times before trying it.

Whatever you do, don't pressure, bribe, or play games to get your child to eat. This will backfire, and he may wind up eating less.

When to Feed Your Child

Toddlers and preschoolers need scheduled meals and snacks. Your child should eat three meals and two to three snacks each day. Make sure to space meals and snacks two to three hours apart to allow your child to become hungry. This way, if he chooses not to eat a meal or snack, it will not be long before the next scheduled meal or snack. Meals should last between 15 and 30 minutes and snacks between 10 and 15 minutes.

Where to Feed Your Child

All food and drink should be consumed at the table or designated location. There is no reason to allow your child to carry food around. This is referred to as grazing, and though it may seem like he is eating a lot, in actuality he is eating less than he should.

Drinks

Serve milk at meals to provide your child with calcium and other vitamins and minerals. At two years of age you can switch your child from whole milk to low-fat milk. Give him only one small serving of juice per day—more than this provides extra sugar and little nutrition. Water is the best choice, especially between meals. Drinking caloric liquids like juice between meals will make your child less hungry at mealtimes.

How Much Is a Serving?

- Children in this age group should eat ¼ to ½ of an adult portion size (example ¼ to ½ sandwich)
- Offer 1 tablespoon of each food for each year of your child's age. For example, offer 2 tablespoons of peas to a two-year-old. If your child is still hungry, offer seconds.

Milk & Dairy

4 servings per day
Serving Size: ½ to ¾ cup

Meat/Protein

3 servings per day
Serving size:

Meat, fish, poultry	1 to 1½ ounces
Eggs	1 egg
Beans	¼ to ½ cup

Peanut Butter	1 to 2 Tbsp
Cottage Cheese	¼ to ½ cup

Fruits & Vegetables

5 servings per day

Serving Size: 2 Tbsp to ½ cup

Juice ¼ to ⅓ cup

Breads, Cereals, & Grains

6 servings per day

Serving Size:

Bread	½ to 1 slice
Cereal	½ to 1 ounce
Oatmeal	¼ to ½ cup
Noodles	¼ to ½ cup
Rice	¼ to ½ cup
Muffin	½ to 1 small
Pancake	½ to 1 small
Roll	½ to 1 small
Biscuit	½ to 1 small
Crackers	2 to 4

Appendix 3

The Food-Chaining Intake Form

Check off foods your child currently eats. If your child previously accepted a food item but no longer eats the food, please circle that item. This will help your feeding team identify patterns in accepted and rejected foods. They may reintroduce a food that your child has successfully eaten in the past. Feel free to write in specific brand names of food items to help with the analysis. Use this form again later in treatment to reevaluate the amounts and types of food your child accepts.

Texture Preferences

- ☐ Crunchy
- ☐ Crisp
- ☐ Smooth
- ☐ Lumpy
- ☐ Uniform lumpy (i.e., cottage cheese)
- ☐ Hard
- ☐ Chewy
- ☐ Mixed consistencies

Taste Preferences

☐ Salty
☐ Sweet
☐ Spicy
☐ Tart
☐ Flavored
☐ Bland

Temperature Preferences

☐ Hot
☐ Warm
☐ Cold
☐ Cool

Appetite

Best time of day to eat ______________________________________

____

Overall description of appetite

☐ Poor
☐ Fair
☐ Good
☐ Varies from day to day

Selective Eating Age of Onset: ____________
Current # Accepted Foods: ________________
Current # Accepted Liquid(s): ____________

Breads

- ☐ Crackers
- ☐ Chips
- ☐ Pretzels
- ☐ Snack mix
- ☐ Bugles
- ☐ Cheese puffs
- ☐ Tostitos/taco chips
- ☐ Taco shells (hard)
- ☐ Flour tortillas
- ☐ Rolls
- ☐ Pizza crusts
- ☐ Hamburger or hot dog buns
- ☐ Bread (white, wheat, rye, potato, rice, gluten-free, pumpernickel, bagels, French bread)
- ☐ Plain bread sticks
- ☐ Garlic bread sticks
- ☐ Texas toast/garlic bread
- ☐ Hot rolls, baked bread, crescent rolls, croissants
- ☐ Biscuits
- ☐ Doughnuts, sweet rolls, cinnamon rolls, caramel rolls
- ☐ Banana bread, pumpkin bread, apple bread, muffins
- ☐ Corn bread
- ☐ Cupcakes
- ☐ Cake, pies, pastries
- ☐ Cheesecake
- ☐ Cookies
- ☐ Other: ______________________________

____

____

Meats

☐ Baked chicken
☐ Fried chicken
☐ Chicken strips
☐ Chicken nuggets
☐ Turkey
☐ Poultry
☐ Fish (fried)
☐ Fish (baked or broiled)
☐ Tuna
☐ Salmon
☐ Beef (steak, roast, deli-style)
☐ Roast
☐ Ribs
☐ Deer
☐ Hamburger
☐ Steak
☐ Ham
☐ Veal
☐ Pork
☐ Sausage
☐ Bacon
☐ Chicken or ham salad
☐ Tuna salad
☐ Meatballs
☐ Hot dogs
☐ Corn dogs
☐ Bologna
☐ Lunch meat
☐ Lil' smokies
☐ Baby food meat sticks
☐ Baby food meats (what types?______________________________)

Nuts

☐ Peanut butter. Specific brands? ______________________________

____

☐ Peanuts

☐ Walnuts

☐ Cashews

☐ Pecans

Potato Products

☐ French fries

☐ Tater tots

☐ Tater rounds

☐ Hash browns

☐ Fried potatoes

☐ Baked potatoes

☐ Potato chips

☐ Potato wedges

☐ Shoestring potato sticks

☐ Mashed potatoes

☐ Mashed potatoes with butter

☐ Mashed potatoes with gravy

☐ Scalloped/au gratin potatoes

☐ Baked sweet potatoes

☐ Candied sweet potatoes

☐ Sweet potato chips

☐ Sweet potato fries

☐ Vegetable chips

☐ Other: ____

____

____

Condiments

☐ Ketchup
☐ Mayonnaise
☐ Miracle Whip
☐ Mustard
☐ Dijon or spicy mustard
☐ Honey mustard
☐ BBQ sauce
☐ A1 Steak Sauce
☐ Chili sauce
☐ Worcestershire sauce
☐ Ranch dressing
☐ Other salad dressings: ________________________________
____
☐ Butter or margarine
☐ Chip dip
☐ Gravy
☐ Other: ____
____
____

Breakfast Foods

☐ Oatmeal
☐ Cream of Wheat
☐ Pop-Tarts (frosted or plain)
☐ Dry cereals
☐ Pancakes
   with fruit
   with syrup
☐ Waffles (homemade)
☐ Waffles (frozen)
☐ French toast

☐ Eggs
  scrambled
  omelet
  fried
  boiled
  poached
  with cheese, vegetables, salsa, chopped meats, etc.
☐ Toast
  with cinnamon and butter
  with jelly
  with apple butter
  with peanut butter
  with honey (after age two)
☐ Breakfast shakes
☐ Yogurt
☐ Go-Gurt (what types?________________________________)
☐ Fresh fruit
☐ Grits

Vegetables
☐ Green beans
☐ Broccoli
☐ Cauliflower
☐ Corn
☐ Squash
☐ Cucumber
☐ Zucchini
☐ Spinach
☐ Carrots
☐ Lettuce
☐ Coleslaw
☐ Cabbage

☐ Sweet potatoes
☐ Tomatoes
☐ Asparagus
☐ Brussels sprouts
☐ Green pepper
☐ Onion
☐ Peas
☐ Salsa
☐ Vegetable baby food (what types?______________________)
☐ Other: ______________________________________
____
____

Liquids

☐ Juice (circle all that apply): orange, cherry, berry, grape, fruit punch, strawberry, strawberry kiwi, cranberry fruit cocktail, white grape, pear, or other: ______________________________
☐ Lemonade
☐ Milk (circle all that apply): whole, 2 percent, skim
☐ Flavored milk (what types?___________________________)
☐ Soda (circle all that apply): cola, lemon-lime, orange, grape, root beer, cream soda. Specific brands:__________________
____
☐ Tea (circle all that apply): sweetened, unsweetened
☐ Milk shakes
☐ Floats
☐ Drinkable yogurt
☐ Water
☐ Caloric supplements (chocolate, vanilla, strawberry, banana cream)
☐ Other: ______________________________________
____
____

Fruits

☐ Apple
☐ Banana
☐ Blueberry
☐ Cantaloupe
☐ Cherry
☐ Grapes
☐ Kiwi
☐ Lemon
☐ Lime
☐ Orange
☐ Pear
☐ Pumpkin
☐ Watermelon
☐ Raisin
☐ Raspberry
☐ Rhubarb
☐ Strawberry
☐ Tangerine
☐ Tomato
☐ Dried fruit

Pasta/Italian-style dishes

☐ Spaghetti
☐ Lasagna
☐ SpaghettiOs/RavioliOs
☐ Casseroles (e.g., Hamburger Helper)
☐ Pizza
☐ Pizza toppings: ____

____

☐ Other: ____

____

- ☐ Rice dishes:____
- ☐ Noodle dishes:______________________________________
- ☐ Couscous

Soups

- ☐ Cheese
- ☐ Cheese and broccoli
- ☐ Cheese and vegetables
- ☐ Chili
- ☐ Stew
- ☐ Vegetable
- ☐ Vegetable beef
- ☐ French onion
- ☐ Egg drop
- ☐ Beef noodle
- ☐ Chicken noodle
- ☐ Chicken and rice
- ☐ Other: ____

____

____

Cheese/Dairy

- ☐ Cheddar
- ☐ American
- ☐ Parmesan
- ☐ Swiss
- ☐ Monterey Jack
- ☐ Mozzarella
- ☐ Colby
- ☐ Cottage cheese
- ☐ Sour cream
- ☐ Yogurt (what types?________________________________)

- ☐ Cool Whip
- ☐ Whipped cream
- ☐ Ice cream (what types? ______________________________)
- ☐ Sherbet (what types? ______________________________)

Fast Foods:

____

____

____

We also analyze favorite and least-favorite foods for patterns and similarities.

Please list your child's favorite foods/liquids:

1.
2.
3.
4.
5.

Please list your child's least-favorite foods/liquids:

1.
2.
3.
4.
5.

What goal foods would you like to see your child eat with the rest of the family?

1.
2.
3.
4.
5.

Are there times when your child eats well?

Is your child taking any medications?

Comments:

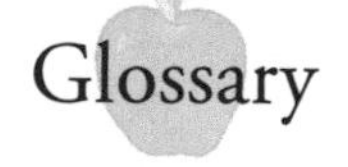

Glossary

Anaphylaxis: A sudden, severe, potentially fatal, systemic allergic reaction that can involve various areas of the body (such as the skin, respiratory tract, GI tract, and cardiovascular system).

Anesthesiologist: A physician specializing solely in anesthesiology to administer anesthetics and related techniques.

Aspiration: The inhalation of food contents into the windpipe and lungs.

Biopsy: The removal of tissue from the body for microscopic examination and diagnosis.

Cervical auscultation: A procedure in which a health-care practitioner listens to the sounds made during the swallow by placing a stethoscope on the neck.

Cleft lip: An abnormal fissure of the lip that failed to close during development.

Cleft palate: Congenital fissure in the median line of the palate which may extend through the uvula, soft palate, and hard palate; cleft lip may also be involved.

Cross-contamination: The transfer of harmful bacteria from one person, object, or place to another.

Dehydration: The excessive loss of fluid from the body due to vomiting, diarrhea, or both.

Delayed gastric emptying: Nerve or muscle damage in the stomach that causes slow digestion and emptying, vomiting, nausea, or bloating. Also called gastroparesis.

Dysphagia: Difficulty swallowing.

Endoscope: A small flexible tube with a light and a lens on the end used to look into the esophagus, stomach, duodenum (first part of the small intestine that connects to the stomach), colon, or rectum.

Endoscopist: A specialist trained in the use of an endoscope.

Epiglottis: The flap that covers the trachea during swallowing so that food does not enter the lungs.

Esophagus: The portion of the digestive canal between the pharynx and stomach.

Esophagitis: Inflammation of the esophagus.

Eustachian tube: The tube that connects the middle ear and the back of the nose, draining the middle ear and regulating air pressure.

Feeding aversion: Extreme food selectivity.

Fiberoptic endoscopic evaluation of the swallow (FEES): A procedure that allows for direct viewing of the swallowing function when regular food materials are eaten by passing a very thin, flexible fiber-optic tube through the nose to obtain a view directly down the throat during swallowing. It is used to help determine the safest position and food texture to maximize nutritional status and eliminate the risk of aspiration and unsafe swallowing.

Food jags: Periods of time when your child will eat only one or two foods.

Fundoplication: A surgical procedure that ties the top of the stomach around the esophagus to prevent reflux.

Fundus: The upper curve of the stomach.

Gastroparesis: Nerve or muscle damage in the stomach that causes slow digestion and emptying, vomiting, nausea, or bloating. Also called delayed gastric emptying.

GERD (Gastroesophageal Reflux Disease): Reflux characterized by frequent vomiting and coughing, choking or gagging whle eating, heartburn or colicky behavior, and regurgitation that causes disease in the GI tract or lungs.

Idiopathic eosinophilic esophagitis (IEE): An allergic inflammatory disease of the esophagus. IEE is usually associated with food or environmental allergens and is most often seen in children. It causes abdominal pain, very painful swallowing and digestion, and vomiting. It can result in children failing to thrive and in weight loss.

Lactation consultant: A health-care professional who specializes in the clinical management of breast-feeding.

Light touch: A diffuse sensation that spreads quickly throughout the body.

Lower esophageal sphincter: The valve at the base of the esophagus that keeps stomach contents (food, acid, and bile) in the stomach, out of the esophagus, and away from the airway.

Malocclusion: When the teeth are not aligned properly.

Mastitis: Inflammation of the breast.

Mitochondrial disorders: Disorders involving the mitochondria or energy units of the cell usually involving the central nervous system and muscles.

Modified barium swallow study: A study completed in radiology to evaluate the swallow function.

Motility: The way food moves through the esophagus, stomach, and intestines.

Obstructive disorders: Obstructive disorders are always associated with airway dysfunction. Examples of obstructive diseases include asthma, chronic bronchitis, and emphysema.

Oral defensiveness: When a baby can't stand having something close to or in his mouth.

Patch test: An allergy test that identifies whether a substance that comes in contact with the skin is causing inflammation of the skin.

Pediatric dietitian: An expert in food and nutrition as they pertain to children.

Pediatric gastroenterologist: A physician that specializes in pediatric specific conditions including liver disease, nutrition, constipation, diarrhea, abdominal pain, nutritional problems, and feeding disorders.

Peristalsis: Wavelike muscle contractions that spread or push food and liquid naturally through the digestive tract.

Pressure touch: Pressure touch receptors are located deep under the skin's surface and have a slow response time. They are responsible for calming the nervous system and allowing us to tolerate approaching touch from others.

Proprioceptive system: The skin pressure and muscle and joint sensory receptors, such as in the joints and spine, that tell us what part of the body is touching the ground as well as what parts of the body are moving.

Pulmonologist: A doctor who specializes in studying and treating diseases of the lungs.

Radiologist: A physician trained in performing and interpreting X-rays.

RAST: A blood test used to determine what a person is allergic to.

Sedation: Intravenous or inhaled medicines to make your child sleepy or fall asleep.

Seizure disorder: A chronic neurological condition characterized by recurrent unprovoked seizures.

Sensory processing disorder: Difficulty in the way the brain takes in, organizes, and uses sensory information, causing a person to have problems interacting effectively in the everyday environment. *Sensory integration dysfunction* is another term for sensory processing disorder.

Skin prick: A test that measures specific IgE attached to cells in the skin important in allergies called "mast" cells.

Spinal cord: The elongated cylindrical portion of the central nervous system that is contained in the spinal canal.

Stereognosis: The ability to perceive the form of an object by using the sense of touch.

Stridor: A noisy type of breathing, happens sometimes when the larynx collapses inward on inspiration in a condition known as laryngomalacia or tracheomalacia (softening of the tracheal rings).

Sudden infant death syndrome (SIDS): The unexpected death during sleep of an apparently healthy infant under one year of age.

Tactile system: Refers to stimulation reaching the central nervous system from receptors in the skin.

Tongue protrusion reflex: An oral reflex seen early in infancy where contact to the tongue causes the tongue to push forward and out of the mouth. This protective reflex helps keep babies safe from choking if a solid object enters their mouths.

Tracheoesophageal fistula: An opening between the trachea and the esophagus.

Vestibular system: The sensory system that provides the dominant input about our movement and orientation in space.

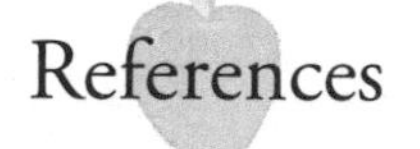

References

Chapter 1

Ferguson, D. D., and A. E. Foxx-Orenstein. 2007. Eosinophilic esophagitis: an update. *Diseases of the Esophagus* 20 (1): 2–8.

Kagalwalla, A. F., and T. Sentongo, S. Ritz, T. Hess, S. P. Nelson, K. M. Emerick, H. Melin-Aldana, B. U. Li. 2006. Effect of six-food elimination diet on clinical and histologic outcomes in eosinophilic esophagitis. *Clinical Gastroenterology and Hepatology.* 4 (9): 1097–1102.

Rudolph, C. D., L. J. Mazur, G. S. Liptak, R. D. Baker, J. T. Boyle, R. B. Colletti, W. T. Gerson, S. L. Werlin. 2001. Guidelines for Evaluation and Treatment of Gastroesophageal Reflux in Infants and Children: Recommendations of the North American Society for Pediatric Gastroenterology and Nutrition. *Journal of Pediatric Gastroenterology & Nutrition* 32 (Suppl. no. 2): S1–S31.

Rudolph, C., and D. T. Link. 2002. Feeding disorders in infants and children. *Pediatric Clinics of North America* 49 (1): S116–S124.

Rudolph, C. D., et al. 2001. Guidelines for evaluation and treatment of gastroesophageal reflux in infants and children. *Journal of Pediatric Gastroenterology & Nutrition* 32 (Suppl. no. 2): 1–31.

Vandenplas, Y. 2005. Gastroesophageal reflux: medical treatment. *Journal of Pediatric Gastroenterology & Nutrition* 41 (Suppl. no. 1): S41–S42.

Chapter 2

Sampson, H. A., S. H. Sicherer, and A. H. Birnbaum, 2001. AGA technical review on the evaluation of food allergy in gastrointestinal disorders. *Gastroenterology* 120: 1026–40.

Bock, S. A. 2003. Diagnostic evaluation. *Pediatrics* 111: 1638–44.

Burks, W. 2003. Skin manifestations of food allergy. *Pediatrics* 111: 1617–24.

Cox, J. H. 1997. *Nutrition Manual for At-Risk Infants and Toddlers.* Chicago: Precept Press.

Duyff, R. L. 2006. *The American Dietetic Association's Complete Food and Nutrition Guide.* Hoboken, NJ: John Wiley & Sons.

Garcia-Careaga, M., and J. Kerner. 2005. Gastrointestinal manifestations of food allergies in pediatric patients. *Nutrition in Clinical Practice* 20: 526–35.

Groh-Wargo, S., M. Thompson, and J. Cox. 2000. *Nutritional Care for High-Risk Newborns.* Chicago: Precept Press.

Joneja, J. V. 2000. *Dietary Management of Food Allergies and Intolerances: A Comprehensive Guide.* Vancouver: J. A. Hall Publications.

Mackay, I., and F. Rosen. 2001. Allergy and allergic diseases. *New England Journal of Medicine* 344 (1): 30–37.

Mackay, I., and F. Rosen. 2001. Allergy and allergic diseases. *New England Journal of Medicine* 344 (2): 109–113.

Mayer, L. 2003. Mucosal immunity. *Pediatrics* 111: 1595–1600.

Mofidi, S. 2003. Nutritional management of pediatric food hypersensitivity. *Pediatrics* 111: 1645–53.

Mohrbacher, N., and J. Stock. 1997. *The Breastfeeding Answer Book.* Schaumburg, IL: La Leche League International.

Munoz-Furlong, A. 2003. Daily coping strategies for patients and their families. *Pediatrics* 111: 1654–61.

Sicherer, S. H. 2003. Clinical aspects of gastrointestinal food allergy in childhood. *Pediatrics* 111: 1609–16.

Sicherer, S., A. Munoz-Furlong, R. Murphy, R. Wood, and H. Sampson. 2003. Symposium: pediatric food allergy. *Pediatrics* 111: 1591–94.

Samour, P. Q., K. Helm, and C. Lang. 1999. *Handbook of pediatric nutrition.* Gaithersburg, MD: Aspen Publishers.

Vanderhoof, J., and R. Young. 2001. Allergic disorders of the gastrointestinal tract. *Current Opinion in Clinical Nutrition and Metabolic Care 4:* 553–56.

Wood, R. A. 2003. The natural history of food allergy. *Pediatrics* 111: 1631–37.

Zieger, R. S. 2003. Food allergen avoidance in the prevention of food allergy in infants and children. *Pediatrics* 111: 1662–71.

Chapter 3

Arvedson, J. C. 1998. Management of pediatric dysphagia. *Otolaryngology Clinics of North America* 31 (3): 453–76.

Arvedson, J. C., and L. Brodsky. 2002. *Management of Feeding and Swallowing Problems: Pediatric Swallowing and Feeding.* Albany, NY: Thomson Learning. 389–468.

Arvedson, J. C., and M. A. Lefton-Greif. 1998. Videofluoroscopic swallow procedures in Pediatrics. In *Pediatric Videofluoroscopic Swallow Studies: A Professional Manual with Caregiver Guidelines.* San Antonio, TX: Communication Skill Builders: The Psychological Corporation. 72–116.

Babbitt, R. L., et al. 1994. Behavioral assessment and treatment of pediatric feeding disorders. *Journal of Developmental and Behavioral Pediatrics* 15: 278–91.

Bisch, E. M., J. A. Logemann, A. W. Rademaker, P. J. Kahrilas, and C. L. Lazarus. 1994. Pharyngeal effects of bolus volume, viscosity, and temperature in patients with dysphagia resulting from neurologic impairment and in normal subjects. *Journal of Speech and Hearing Research* 37: 1041–59.

Burklow, K. A., A. Phelps, J. Schultz, K. McConnell, and C. Rudolph. 1998. Classifying complex pediatric feeding disorders. *Journal of Pediatric Gastroenterology and Nutrition* 27 (2): 143–47.

Clark, H. M. 2003. Neuromuscular treatment for speech and swallowing: a tutorial. *American Journal of Speech-Language Pathology* 12: 400–15.

Dodds, W. J. 1989. Physiology of swallowing. *Dysphagia* 3: 171–78.

Cherney, L. 1994. *Clinical management of dysphagia in adults and children.* Gaithersburg, MD: Aspen Publishers.

Fraker, C., and L. Walbert. 2001. *Evaluation and treatment of pediatric feeding disorders: From NICU to childhood.* Austin, TX: ProEd Publishers.

Glass, R., and L. Wolf. 1992. *Feeding and swallowing disorders in infancy.* Tucson: Therapy Skill Builders.

Kedesdy, J., and K. Budd. 1998. *Childhood feeding disorders: Biobehavioral assessment and intervention.* Baltimore: Paul H. Brookes Publishing Co.

Leder, S. B., and D. E. Karas. 2000. Fiberoptic endoscopic evaluation of swallowing in the pediatric population. *The Laryngoscope* 110: 1132–36.

Morris, S. E., and M. D. Klein. 1987. *Pre-feeding skills.* Tucson: Therapy Skill Builders.

Neifert, M., R. Lawrence, and J. Seatcat. 1995. Nipple confusion: toward a formal definition. *Journal of Pediatrics* l, 126:S125–29.

Newman, L. 2000. Optimal care patterns in pediatric patients with dysphagia. *Seminars in Speech and Language* 21 (4): 281–91.

Newman L., C. Keckley, M. Peterson, and A. Hammer. 2001. Swallowing function and medical diagnosis in infants suspected of dysphagia. *Pediatrics* 108 (6):E106

Rozin, P. 1996. Sociocultural influences on human food selection. In *Why We Eat What We Eat: The Psychology of Eating.* Washington, D.C.: American Psychological Association. 233–63.

Ruark, J. L., G. H. McCullough, R. Peters, and C. A. Moore. 2002. Bolus consistency and swallowing in children and adults. *Dysphagia* 17: 24–33.

Ruark, J. L., C. E. Mills, and R. A. Muenchen. 2003. Effects of bolus volume and consistency on multiple swallow behavior in children and adults. *Journal of Medical Speech-Language Pathology* 11 (4): 213–26.

Chapter 4

Anzalone, M. E. 2004. Sensory strategies and self-regulation in young children: strategies for assessment and intervention. *The Young Child with Special Needs.* Nashville: Contemporary Forums.

Bundy, A., S. Lane, and E. Murray (eds.). 1991. *Sensory Integration Theory and Practice.* Philadelphia: F. A. Davis.

Frontera, W. R., D. M. Dawson, and D. M. Slovik. 1999. *Exercise in Rehabilitative Medicine.* Champaign, IL: Human Kinetics.

Gisel, E. G. 1998. Chewing cycles in two- to eight-year-old normal children: a developmental profile." *American Journal of Occupational Therapy* 42(1), 40–46.

Glass, R., and L. Wolf. 1992. *Feeding and Swallowing Disorders in Infancy.* Tucson: Therapy Skill Builders.

Hanschu, Bonnie. 1999. *Evaluation and Treatment of Sensory Processing Disorders.* Florida: Developmental Concepts.

Kisner, C., and L. A. Colby. 1996. *Therapeutic Exercise: Foundations and Techniques.* 3rd ed. Philadelphia: F. A. Davis.

Kranowitz, C. S. 1998. *The Out-of-Sync Child: Recognizing and Coping with Sensory Integration Dysfunction.* New York: Perigee.

McCormack, G. L. 1996. The Rood approach to treatment of neuromuscular dysfunction. In L. W. Pedretti (ed.), *Occupational Therapy: Practice Skills for Physical Dysfunction.* St. Louis: Mosby. 377–99.

Williamson, G., and M. Anzalone. 2001. *Sensory Integration and Self-Regulation in Infants and Toddlers: Helping Very Young Children Interact with Their Environment.* Washington, D.C.: Zero to Three Publishers.

Chapter 5

Birch, L., and J. Fisher. 1998. Development of eating behaviors among children and adolescents. *Pediatrics* 101: 539–49.

Birch, L. 1990. Development of food acceptance patterns. *Developmental Psychology* 26: 515–19.

Birch, L., and J. Fisher. 1995. Appetite and eating behavior in children. *The Pediatric Clinics of North America: Pediatric Nutrition.* 42(4): 931–53.

Birch, L., and J. Fisher. 1996. The role of experience in the development of children's eating behavior. In *Why We Eat What We Eat: The Psychology of Eating.* Washington, D.C.: American Psychological Association. 113–41.

Crist, W., and A. Napier-Phillips. 2001. Mealtime behaviors of young children: A comparison of normative and clinical data. Feeding strategies for older infants and toddlers. *Developmental and Behavioral Pediatrics* 22: 279–86.

Duffy, V. B., and L. M. Bartoshuk. 1996. Sensory factors in feeding. In *Why We Eat What We Eat: The Psychology of Eating.* Washington, D.C.: American Psychological Association. 145–71.

Mennella, J. A., and G. K. Beauchamp. 1996. The early development of human flavor preferences. In *Why We Eat What We Eat: The Psychology of Eating.* Washington, D.C.: American Psychological Association. 83–112.

O'Brien, M. 1996. Child-rearing difficulties reported by parents of infants and toddlers. *Journal of Pediatric Psychology* 21: 433–46.

Satter, E. 2000. *Child of Mine: Feeding with Love and Good Sense.* Palo Alto, CA: Bull Publishing Company.

Chapter 6

Crook, C. K., and L. P. Lipsitt. 1976 Neonatal nutritive sucking: Effects of taste stimulation on sucking and heart rate. *Child Development* 47: 518–29.

Desour, J. A., O. Maller, and R. E. Turner. 1973. Taste in acceptance of sugars by human infants. *The Journal of Comparative and Physiological Psychology* 84: 496.

Ding, R., J. A. Logemann, C. R. Larson, and A. W. Rademaker. 2003. The effects of taste and consistency on swallow physiology in younger and older healthy individuals: A surface electromyographic study." *Journal of Speech-Language and Hearing Research* 46 (4): 977–89.

Mennella, J. A., and G. K. Beauchamp 1997. The ontogeny of human flavor perception. In G. K. Beauchamp and L. Bartoshuk (eds.) *Tasting and Smelling.* San Diego, CA: Academic Press. 199–221.

Pelletier, C. A., and H. T. Lawless. 2003. Effect of citric acid–sucrose mixtures on swallowing in neurogenic oropharyngeal dysphagia. *Dysphagia* 18: 231–41.

Pinnington, L., and J. Hegarty. 2000. Effects of consistent food presentation on oral-motor skill development acquisition in children with severe neurological impairment. *Dysphagia* 15: 213–23.

Reau, N. R., Y. D. Senturia, S. A. Lebailly, and K. K. Christoffel. 1996. Infant and toddler feeding patterns and problems: normative data and new direction. *Journal of Developmental and Behavioral Pediatrics* 17 (3): 149–53.

Chapter 7

Fraker, C., and L. Walbert. 2001. *Evaluation and Treatment of Pediatric Feeding Disorders: From NICU to Childhood.* Austin, TX: ProEd Publishers.

Hulme, J. B., J. Shaver, S. Acher, L. Mullette, and C. Eggert. 1987. Effects of adaptive seating devices on eating and drinking in children with multiple handicaps. *American Journal of Occupational Therapy,* 41(2):81-9.

Mathew, O. P., M. Belan, and C. Thoppil. 1992 Sucking patterns of neonates during bottle feeding: comparison of different nipple units. *American Journal of Perinatology 9*: 265–69.

Pinnington, L., and J. Hegarty. 2000. Effects of consistent food presentation on oral-motor skill development acquisition in children with severe neurological impairment. *Dysphagia* 15: 213–23.

Rudolph, C., and D. T. Link. 2002. Feeding disorders in infants and children. *Pediatric Clinics of North America* 49(1): S116–S124.

Rudolph, C. D., et al. 2001. Guidelines for evaluation and treatment of gastroesophageal reflux in infants and children. *Journal of Pediatric Gastroenterology and Nutrition* 32 (Suppl. no. 2): 1–31.

Chapter 8

Garvey, J. 2002. Diet in autism and associated disorders. *Journal of Family Health Care* 12: 34–38.

Gisel, E. G. 1994. Oral-motor skills following sensorimotor intervention in the moderately eating-impaired child with cerebral palsy. *Dysphagia* 9: 180–92.

Helfrich-Miller, K. R., K. L. Rector, and J. A. Straka. 1986. Dysphagia: its treatment in the profoundly retarded patient with cerebral palsy. *Archives of Physical Medicine and Rehabilitation* 67: 520–25.

Hulme, J. B., J. Shaver, S. Acher, L. Mullette, and C. Eggert. 1987. Effects of adaptive seating devices on eating and drinking in children with multiple handicaps *American Journal of Occupational Therapy,* 41(2):81-9.

Larnert, G., and O. Ekberg. 1995. Positioning improves oral and pharyngeal swallow function in children with cerebral palsy. *Acta Paediatrica* 84: 689–92.

Morris, S. E. 1989. Development of oral-motor skills in the neurologically impaired child receiving non-oral feedings. *Dysphagia* 3: 135–54.

Neilson, P. D., G. Andrews, B. E. Guitar, and P. T. Quinn. 1979. Tonic stretch reflexes in lip, tongue, and jaw muscles. *Brain Research* 178: 311–27.

Reilly, S., and D. Skuse. 1992. Characteristics and management of feeding problems of young children with cerebral palsy. *Developmental Medicine and Child Neurology* 34: 379–88.

Rogers, B., J. Arvedson, G. Buck, P. Smart, and M. Msall. 1994. Characteristics of dysphagia in children with cerebral palsy. *Dysphagia* 9: 69–73.

Rudolph, C., and D. T. Link. 2002. Feeding disorders in infants and children. *Pediatric Clinics of North America* 49 (1). S116–S124.

Rudolph, C. D., et al. 2001. Guidelines for evaluation and treatment of gastroesophageal reflux in infants and children. *Journal of Pediatric Gastroenterology and Nutrition* 32 (Suppl. no. 2): 1–31.

Schwarz, S., J. Corredor, J. Fisher-Medina, J. Cohen, and S. Rabinowitz. 2001. Diagnosis and treatment of feeding disorders in children with developmental disabilities. *American Academy of Pediatrics* 108 (3): 671–76.

Shaker, C. S. 1990. Nipple feeding premature infants: A different perspective. *Neonatal Network* 8 (5): 9–17.

Shivpuri, C. R., et al. 1983. Decreased ventilation in preterm infants during oral feeding. *Journal of Pediatrics* 103 (2): 285–89.

Tcheremenska, A. R., and E. G. Gisel. 1994. Use of substitute food textures for standard eating assessment in children with cerebral palsy and children without disabilities. *The American Journal of Occupational Therapy* 48 (7): 626–32.

Vandenberg, K. A. 1990. Nippling management of the sick neonate in the ICU: the disorganized feeder. *Neonatal Network* 9 (1): 9–16.

Vazquez, J. L. 1999. Feeding difficulties in the first days of life: findings on upper gastrointestinal series and the role of the videofluoroscopic swallowing study. *Pediatric Radiology* 29 (12): 894–96.

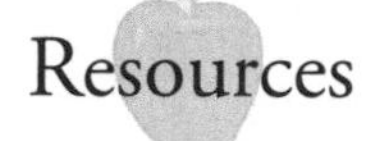

Resources

For conferences for professionals on food chaining and feeding disorders in infants and children, contact www.cepauniversity.com for online registration.

For conferences for parent groups, contact us at www.preemietalk.org.

To schedule an appointment with Cheri, Laura, and Sibyl:
The Center for Selective Eating and Pediatric Feeding Disorders
Koke Mill Medical Center
3132 Old Jacksonville Road
Springfield, Illinois 62704
Phone: (217) 862-0400
Fax: (217) 862-0440

Sibyl also sees patients at:
The SIU School of Medicine
P.O. Box 19658
301 North 8th Street
Springfield, Illinois 62794
Phone: (217) 545-0702

Dr. Fishbein sees patients at:
Children's Memorial Hospital
2300 Children's Plaza (Lincoln and Fullerton)
Chicago, Illinois 60614
Phone: (800) KIDS-DOC

Organizations:
American Academy of Pediatrics
141 Northwest Point Boulevard
Elk Grove Village, Illinois 60007-1098
Phone: (847) 434-4000
Fax: (847) 434-8000
Web site: www.aap.org

The American Dietetic Association
216 West Jackson Boulevard
Chicago, Illinois 60606
Web site: www.eatright.org

American Speech Language and Hearing Association (ASHA)
10801 Rockville Pike
Rockville, Maryland 20852
Toll free: (800) 638-8255
Fax: (240) 333-4705
Web site: www.asha.org

Celiac Sprue Association
P.O. Box 31700
Omaha, Nebraska 68131-0700
Toll free: (877) CSA-4-CSA
Phone: (402) 558-0600
Web site: www.csaceliacs.org

Food and Drug Administration (FDA)
Center for Food Safety and Applied Nutrition
Outreach and Information Center
5100 Paint Branch Parkway HFS-555

College Park, Maryland 20740-3835
Toll free: (888) 723-3366
Web site: www.fda.gov

Food and Nutrition Information Center
National Agricultural Library
U.S. Department of Agriculture
10301 Baltimore Avenue
Beltsville, Maryland 20705
Web site: http://fnic.nal.usda.gov

La Leche League International
Web site: www.lalecheleague.org
If you don't have access to a computer, look in your local telephone directory. Many La Leche League groups have listings in the white or yellow pages. Some are also listed in the free "blue" pages for nonprofit organizations. If there is no listing under "La Leche League," look under headings labeled "breast-feeding" or "lactation." In some places La Leche League will be listed under "community resources" or "women's health." You can also call 1-800-LALECHE or (847) 519-7730. The second number provides access to an automated system for finding LLL leaders in the United States by entering a local zip code. In Canada, telephone 1-800-665-4324, or (514) LALECHE for a French-speaking leader.

The National Dairy Council
Web site: www.nationaldairycouncil.org

These two organizations offer information on pediatric GI disorders such as GERD and can also help you locate a pediatric gastroenterologist:

North American Society for Pediatric Gastroenterology, Hepatology, and Nutrition (NASPGHAN)
P.O. Box 6
Flourtown, Pennsylvania 19031
Phone: (215) 233-0808
Fax: (215) 233-3918
E-mail: naspghan@naspghan.org
Web site: www.naspghan.org

Children's Digestive Health and Nutrition Foundation (CDHNF)
Toll-free: 800-344-8888
Web site: www.cdhnf.org

Recommended Web sites:
www.theautismlife.com
This site is packed with teaching ideas, product guides, recipes, interviews with professionals, photos, and stories of encouragement for parents of children with autistic spectrum disorder.

Cosmeo Web site: www.cosmeo.com
This site offers academic, development, and video learning for children grades K-12.

Recommended Chemistry/Food Web sites:
These Web sites provide great ideas for helping young children understand very basic concepts about food and helping older children understand more complex ones. Some of the experiments on these Web sites are more applicable to older children, but they can easily be adapted for a younger child. The most important thing to remember is to keep things simple and fun. These Web sites are just a few of the hundreds out there on the Internet when it comes to food, food science, and ways to incorporate food items and concepts into your lives. We encourage you to explore.

http://www.scholastic.com/schoolage/activities/k_2/kitchensci.htm
http://personal.cfw.com/~rollinso/SciFood.html
http://chemistry.about.com/od/homeexperiments/
http://www.chatham.edu/pti/Kitchen_Chem/BCleveland_01.htm
http://www.foodscience.psu.edu/outreach/fun_food_science.html
http://www.clubmom.com/display/245307
http://homeschooling.gomilpitas.com/explore/chemistry.htm
http://homeschooling.gomilpitas.com/explore/chemistryfood.htm

Food Allergy Resources:
American Academy of Allergy, Asthma, and Immunology
555 East Wells Street
Suite 1100
Milwaukee, Wisconsin 53202-3823
Phone: (414) 272-6071
Patient Information and Physician Referral Line: (800) 822-2762

E-mail: info@aaaai.org
Web site: www.aaaai.org

Asthma and Allergy Foundation of America
1233 20th Street NW
Suite 402
Washington, D.C. 20036
Toll free: (800) 727-8462
E-mail: info@aafa.org
Web site: www.aafa.org

Food Allergy and Anaphylaxis Network
11781 Lee Jackson Hwy., Suite 160
Fairfax, Virginia 22033-3309
Phone: (800) 929-4040
Fax: (703) 691-2713
E-mail: faan@foodallergy.org
Web site: www.foodallergy.org

The following books offer good information and advice for living with and cooking for food allergies:

Barber, Marianne. *The Parent's Guide to Food Allergies: Clear and Complete Advice from the Experts on Raising Your Food-Allergic Child.* New York: Owl Books, 2001.

Kidder, Beth, and Harold Friedman. *The Milk Free Kitchen: Living Well without Dairy Products.* New York: Owl Books, 1991.

Muñoz-Furlong, Anne (ed.). *The Food Allergy News Cookbook: A Collection of Recipes from Food Allergy News and Members of the Food Allergy Network.* New York: Wiley, 1998.

Eden Foods
701 Tecumseh Road
Clinton, Michigan 49236
Toll free: (888) 424-333
E-mail: info@edenfoods.com
Web site: www.edenfoods.com

Ener-G-Foods
5960 First Avenue South
P.O. Box 84487
Seattle, Washington 98124-5787
Toll free: (800) 331-5222
Fax: (206) 764-3398
E-mail: customerservice@ener-g.com
Web site: www.ener-g.com

The Gluten Free Pantry
glutenfree.com
P.O. Box 840
Glastonbury, Connecticut 06033
Inquiries, Orders & Customer Service: (800) 291-8386
Consumer Information & Education: (860) 633-3826
Fax: (450) 963-0137
Web site: www.glutenfree.com

Barbara's Bakery
c/o WorldPantry.com, Inc.
601 22nd Street
San Francisco, California 94107
Toll-free: (866) 972-6879
Phone: (415) 401-0080
Fax: (415) 401-0087
Web site: www.worldpantry.com/cgibin/ncommerce/ExecMacro/barbarasbakery/home.d2w/report

Recommended Reading

Cox, Janice H. *Nutrition Manual for At-Risk Infants and Toddlers.* Chicago, IL: Precept Press, 1997.

Groh-Wargo, Sharon, Melody Thompson, and Janice Cox. *Nutritional Care for High-Risk Newborns.* Chicago, IL: Precept Press, 2000.

Kranowitz, Carol Stock. *The Out-of-Sync Child: Recognizing and Coping with Sensory Integration Dysfunction.* New York: Perigee, 2005.

Acknowledgments

We would like to thank our parents and our families, Margie, Katie, Ellie, Joey, Patricia, Chuck, Emma, Cory, Justin, Lily, Simon, Brett, Gianna, Randy, and Luke. You are our joy and God has blessed us with all of you. Thank you to Jennifer Chalekson, RD, Chris Mogren, RN, and Cheryl Swenny, psychologist, who make up the rest of our little feeding-team family. We love and treasure your friendship and loyalty. Special thanks to Alicia Hart, Ewan Nees, and Stacey Vitale, CCC/SLP, for the contributions you made to this project and to our lives.

Countless nurses, therapists, and physicians have contributed to our knowledge and work over the years; we thank you for your generous spirits and caregiver hearts. We would also like to thank Sue McCloskey and Shannon Cole Barker, OTR/L, for their hours of work on this project and for sharing their gifts with us. We so appreciate everyone at Avalon Publishing, especially Matthew Lore and Katie McHugh, for believing in and supporting this project. Thanks to Vince Kunkemueller for guiding the book through the production process, Donna Stonecipher for the copyediting, Ann Kirchner for the proofreading, and Andrew Newman for the wonderful cover design.

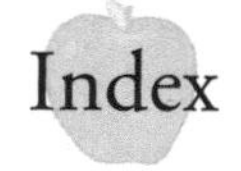

Index